3.16.79

Contents

Acknowledgments   9

The Doctor Wants to See Me   13

Tears and Questions   22

A Ray of Hope   31

Love Tested   38

I Need Jesus   48

Another Mother Reaches Out   56

My Life Is Changing   67

A View of the Future   78

An Unrealistic Dream   87

One Beautiful Reason   99

Lessons I Needed to Learn   111

Would You Believe I Have a Jealousy Problem?   121

People, Not God, Put Labels on People   133

A Time of Victories   145

Staying Up With the Down's Syndrome Child   161

Lorie

Lorie:

a story of hope

Mary Ann Cobb

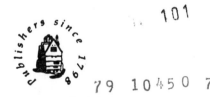

Publishers since 1798

Thomas Nelson Publishers
Nashville ● New York

All rights reserved under International and Pan-American Conventions. Published in Nashville, Tennessee, by Thomas Nelson Inc., Publishers and simultaneously in Don Mills, Ontario, by Thomas Nelson & Sons (Canada) Limited. Manufactured in the United States of America.

Library of Congress Cataloging in Publication Data

Cobb, Mary Ann.
  Lorie : a story of hope.

  Bibliography: p. 179
  1. Down's syndrome—Biography. 2. Christian life—
1960-   3. Cobb, Lorie Lynn, 1974-
RJ506.D68C6   362.7'8'30926   78-20951
ISBN 0-8407-5677-1

I dedicate this book to our very special child, Lorie Lynn Cobb, who brightens our lives and whose coming brought us to Jesus Christ, our Savior—for all He is doing through her in our lives to shape us into what He desires us to be and for the other people who have come to call on the Lord because she has touched their lives.

2065231

Acknowledgments

I want to thank all the people who have helped this book come about:

To Donald, my husband, who has been my greatest supporter and constant encourager.

To Cris Holl, my best friend, who has helped with this book since its conception. Her help in corrections and typing are invaluable.

To Marge Green, an author in her own right, who helped with grammar.

To the professionals in our lives, who let me tell about them: Dr. Lucille Poor, Dante Cicchetti, Linda Manns, Chris Byroads, and Rae-Ann Anderson.

And to my friends and relatives who allowed me to tell you their stories.

It is my hope our story will glorify Jesus Christ and show His great love for all of us!

The Doctor Wants to See Me

For He has not despised nor abhorred the affliction of the afflicted; Neither has He hidden His face from him; But when he cried to Him for help, He heard (Ps. 22:24).

One day four years ago our even-keeled world was turned topsy-turvy. Oh, we didn't know it when the day started out, but before it was over, an event occurred that changed the course of our lives.

The day began as most other days do, except it was Christmas Eve. We had planned our Christmas to be a quiet one this year, with only our immediate family. The day did not end quietly; Donald took me to the hospital, and we became parents of a small baby girl at 11:27 P.M.

On Christmas Day, 1974, as we held our new daughter and marveled over how lucky we were to now have both a boy and a girl, Don and I joked about Lorie's early arrival. Don brought Kevin, our four-year-old son, to see his new sister during children's visiting hours. He peeked at her through the nursery windows and exclaimed, "She's so small!" Then, as if he had forgotten about her, he asked, "When are you coming home, Mommy?"

Our first day of basking in the enjoyment of our new daughter went by quickly, and evening began as darkness started hiding the daylight.

Don looked at his watch. "Honey, I'm going to have to go if I'm going to pick up your sister at the bus depot." I watched him leave.

Peggy, my sister, had agreed to come and take care of Kevin. Mom and Dad had planned to come, but Lorie blew our plans and surprised us by arriving two weeks early.

The nurse's aide had just placed my supper tray before me, and I was about to bite into a large hamburger when an older nurse came to tell me that the pediatrician would like to meet me in the mothers' lounge.

"Right now?"

"Yes. Here, let me take your tray and keep your supper warm."

I put down the hamburger, not even one bite taken, and handed the tray over. The nurse whisked it away, leaving me to the silence of the room. *Why did the doctor want to see me in the mothers' lounge? Why didn't he want to come to my room to talk to me?* When I had Kevin, the doctor came into my room to tell me how healthy our baby was. I wondered if meeting with the doctor in the mothers' lounge meant that something was wrong with my baby.

I wasn't finding out anything this way, so I put on my slippers and housecoat and went to keep the appointment with the doctor.

Oh, how I wished Donald were there! If only the doctor had arrived a few minutes earlier! And I hoped I

14

would be able to remember correctly what the doctor would tell me, so I could relay it to Donald.

The mothers' lounge was deserted and dark. I switched on the light, and thumbed through a magazine, but I couldn't concentrate on it. What if the doctor told me bad news concerning Lorie? What would we do? My mind went on and on, churning up troubling thoughts.

The circumstances in Kevin's and Lorie's births were different; something was definitely up! Little did I know that Don and I were about to enter the biggest problem and adjustment process of our eight years of marriage.

The past year had already been one of many adjustments. Don had changed jobs (requiring a one hundred and twenty-mile move to a suburb of Minneapolis, Minnesota), and I had quit my job of five years to become a full-time homemaker. We had been in the Twin Cities only six weeks when our daughter was born.

Lorie was a tiny one, tipping the scale at four pounds thirteen-and-a-half ounces, and measuring eighteen inches in length. She had a small, round face framed with light brown hair. I had wondered why she was so small, but then brushed the thought from my mind. She looked perfect to me.

Waiting for the doctor was murder. By now I had thought up all kinds of things our baby could have: a bad heart, malfunctioning kidneys, and a host of other health problems. It seemed almost unbearable. I felt like a person waiting for the jury to come in with the verdict. Oh, how I wished the doctor would hurry so we could get this over with.

"Mrs. Cobb," the doctor said, breaking the silence, "I've just finished examining your baby."

"What did you find out?" I hesitantly asked him.

"My examination indicates that your daughter is Mongoloid."

Mongoloid! Aren't they the weird-looking babies in institutions? (Later I would be told that the medical term is Down's Syndrome.)

"How can you know? She's just newborn— why—what?"

The doctor took a deep breath and said, "Your daughter was born with a chromosome error. She has forty-seven chromosomes in every cell instead of forty-six as normal people have. We don't know why this happens, but something goes wrong in the blue print and the baby doesn't form right."

This is a nightmare! I'm going to wake up— aren't I?

"They are doing research to find out why, but so far they haven't come across a definite answer," he continued.

"What does this mean? I don't know anything about Mongoloid babies!" I was going through the motions of asking him questions. It seemed as if I were someone else; I was trying not to feel anything.

"First, she will be mentally retarded. She will have poor muscle tone, hypotonia, so she will be slower at doing things like crawling. There is nothing we can do to change it. This is a permanent condition."

"How can you know for sure? Our baby's only a few hours old!"

"By various signs. She has the small curved finger, wide split between the first and second toes, the shape of her eyes, her small low-set ears, poor muscle tone, and the tongue that sticks out."

"She doesn't look it!" I protested. "I have the small curved finger." I wanted to talk him out of what he was trying to tell me.

"We may all have some of these signs, but it is the

16

combination of signs and poor muscle tone that leads me to suspect this condition."

"Do you know for sure?" I questioned.

"No, not absolutely. That will have to be done with karyotyping."

"What's that?"

"It's a blood test where we draw some of her blood. We study it on a slide when the cell is in the dividing stage, and by pairing the cell, we will be able to see for sure if she has an extra chromosome."

Oh, my God, what are we going to do now? His words were sinking in, and tears started rolling down my cheeks.

"I'm sorry," the doctor's voice cracked. "I wish there were something we could do."

This is true! We have a baby handicapped with something I never would have dreamed of in a million years!

"Do you have any questions?" he asked.

"No." I couldn't grasp anything more.

I watched the doctor leave. He was no doubt glad to have this difficult task over with.

Our daughter—Mongoloid—why? I don't understand! What are we going to do? The tears became a torrent as I realized what the doctor had told me.

I bolted out of the lounge and started running toward my room. I wanted to fling myself across the bed and cry and cry and cry.

Jan, my roommate, was sitting on the edge of her bed when I ran in. "Mary Ann, what's the matter?" she asked.

"Something is wrong with our baby! She's Mongoloid."

Jan put her arm around my shoulder. I was glad she was there to help ease the hurt. I began to tell her what the doctor had told me only a few minutes before. I could see that she felt some of the hurt I was feeling.

"Oh, Jan, it was so perfect today, and now it seems as if the rug has been pulled out from under me." I had stopped crying, but deep down the hurt was nearly unbearable.

It was seven o'clock now, and I lay in bed with a million questions. What will it be like taking care of her? Will I be able to do it?

"Mary Ann," my girl friend Marie said as she entered the room. "I peeked at your baby—she is so cute and so small."

When she handed me a baby present, she noticed that my eyes were red and swollen. "Mary Ann, what in the world is the matter?"

"The doctor just told me something is wrong with our baby."

"What?" Marie's happy look changed quickly to a sad one.

"She's Mongoloid!"

Slowly, I told her the sad story.

It was not until I was home from the hospital that I realized what Marie had done for me and how she had felt that night. After I told her the sad news, she decided she couldn't leave me until Don came back. She kept from breaking down in front of me, as she didn't want to upset me, but when she left she put her head down on the steering wheel and cried. She felt sad and torn apart, realizing our grief, and she tried to understand why it had happened to us.

Marie left when my sister came into the room—Don had sent her ahead, while he tended her two sons in the lobby.

"You know?" she asked when she saw my red, swollen eyes.

"What do you mean?" I was stunned by her question.

"Don told me about Lorie on the way over here. The doctor told him last night."

"Why didn't Don tell me?"

I didn't understand why he had kept it from me, and I was surprised he knew; he had hidden it so well from me all day. Don had come in the morning, donned his green paper gown, and promptly gotten his daughter out of the nursery. He had picked her up carefully and admired and cuddled her during the time he was there.

Come to think of it, he had kept asking me if the doctor had come. I couldn't imagine why he kept asking, as I doubted that a doctor would come on Christmas Day.

I wanted to see Don and asked my sister to get him. I waited impatiently until he arrived. As soon as I saw him, the tears poured down my cheeks again.

"You found out—how?" Don questioned. Concern showed on his face.

"The doctor told me in the mothers' lounge right after you left. I never dreamed anything was wrong! How did you find out? Why didn't you tell me?"

Don sat on the edge of the bed and gathered me in his arms—we needed each other. How comforting to feel his strong arms around me. I felt warm and secure. We were facing this together.

"When I was waiting in the hall, while you were getting settled in recovery, I saw the doctor. He had a worried look on his face, and I asked him to level with me. I knew something must be wrong. He wanted to tell you right away, but I said no. I wanted to wait until the pediatrician had looked at the baby and was pretty sure. I didn't want to upset you and then have the pediatrician say it wasn't true."

Suddenly I understood why the doctor had come in to see me in the recovery room. Usually, after the baby is delivered, you don't see a doctor until the next day.

Lorie

The doctor had held my hand, and with a concerned look had told me: "I'm calling in a pediatrician to look over your baby. Now, it's not because she is in serious condition and needs immediate surgery or anything, but I want to have her checked over as a precaution."

Why hadn't I noticed more that night? Maybe I had known it was more than normal concern but had blocked it out of my mind because I really didn't want to believe it.

"Don, I wish you would have let my obstetrician tell me. It would have been better than a strange doctor telling me while I was alone."

"Oh, honey," he said sadly, "I never meant for you to be told the way you were."

"How did you carry this burden alone?" I asked. I just couldn't imagine how he had managed to keep it from me.

"It was hard—I didn't sleep much last night. I tried to call Rita [a friend of ours who is a nurse], so she could tell me more. Wouldn't you know she wasn't home?"

Tears were streaming down Don's cheeks. "I don't care what's wrong with her; she's ours, and we are going to take her home and do the best we can with her!" he said.

I loved him so much at that moment.

"Oh, Don, why us? Will I be able to cope with this? Why did God let this happen to us?"

"I don't know why He let it happen." I could sense Don's deep sadness and hurt, too. "We'll manage together; somehow we'll do it."

"Do you think God is punishing us for our sins?" I couldn't imagine why God would let innocent children suffer.

"I don't think so."

"But why? And why us?"

Isn't it funny? All of our lives we thought that things like this happened only to others.

"Don, what if no one wants to know us or cares about our baby because she is different?" I could see us going home and no one wanting to hold her because she was different.

"Oh, honey," Don tried to reassure me, "I don't think people will feel that way."

"Don, I won't be able to stand it if no one wants to hold our baby!"

"It doesn't matter; we love her. I don't know what the future will bring, but she will have us." To Don there was no other solution, except taking her home and loving her.

"I guess I'd better go and take Peg and the boys home. I'll see you tomorrow when I can." His voice showed a desire to stay with me, and how I wished he could.

"Come as soon as you can tomorrow," I pleaded.

"I will; you know I will." Don's voice calmed me.

We clung to each other for a couple of minutes and then he was off, taking long, striding steps.

A nurse's aide tried to cheer me up. She told me that she would bring the book *Angel Unaware* by Dale Evans for me to read.

I was glad to go to sleep that night and took the first sleeping pill I'd ever taken in my life. I wanted to rest—maybe things would look better tomorrow.

Tears and Questions

How happy are those who know what sorrow means, for they will be given courage and comfort! (Matt. 5:4).*

When I woke up, the room was still dark. I rolled over to look at the clock on the bedside table. Five A.M. Why did I wake up this early? I lay a couple of minutes in the quiet of the room before the memories of the last night's events rushed through my mind.

I started crying. *Something is wrong with the darling baby girl I had held and loved immediately.*

It's hard to describe the feelings I had at that moment. I felt hurt, mad, confused, and I didn't know what life was going to be like with her. I was afraid and mixed-up. Most of all, I didn't understand why God had let this happen to us!

*J. B. Phillips, *The New Testament in Modern English*, revised edition. ©J. B. Phillips 1958, 1960, 1972. Used by permission of Macmillan Publishing Co, Inc.

The future scared me, and I hardly knew anything about Mongolism. What would be involved in taking care of her?

It isn't fair! How can I cope? Oh, I just don't understand why!

I could hear the sounds of morning activity outside the door of our room. Another day was starting. A nurse popped thermometers into our mouths. Life has a way of going on no matter what has happened, and I numbly managed to go through the morning routines.

"Mary Ann, let's go and get our babies," Jan suggested after we had eaten breakfast.

"All right." I hadn't held or fed Lorie since just before the doctor had told me. I had been too upset afterward to tend to her.

Jan and I went to the nursery and asked the nurse if we could have our babies.

"Sure," she answered, slamming the door shut on a cabinet. I saw Lorie jump; in fact, she was the only baby who really noticed it. At least she has good hearing, I thought.

Our babies were in clear plastic beds that were placed on top of little carts with wheels. We rolled our babies back to the room. We could keep our babies as much or as little as we wanted them, except during regular visiting hours.

I picked Lorie up—she was so light. She moved her little arms and legs and looked around a bit. She was such a pretty baby and didn't look any different from the other babies. I couldn't imagine that in time she would look different and that people would notice.

She seemed content to lie in my arms. I lay back in my bed holding her closely. I did love her—she was my baby.

After awhile I unwrapped her receiving blanket and looked for the signs that the doctor had told me were there. Every one of them was there, just as he had said. I hadn't noticed them before.

"She won't seem different at first, but at about six months of age, she will start to lag behind," a nurse had told me after Don had left the night before.

I looked at my little daughter fast asleep in my arms and wondered what life would be like for her. Would she realize her handicap? Would it make it hard for her in a world where a premium is placed on being normal? Would she be sad, or would she be happy? Oh, baby, I thought as I gazed down at her, there is just so much I don't know about you. I'm going to have to learn.

As I was enjoying the quiet time with my baby, a middle-aged woman came into the room. She was the social worker at the hospital.

"I came by to see if I can be of any help to you," she said, and sat down in a nearby chair.

"I had a little girl who was born with chromosome damage, too. Her chromosome errors were in the fourteenth and fifteenth chromosomes. Your baby's chromosome error is in the twenty-first chromosomes."

"What does that mean?" I anxiously questioned.

"Well, whichever chromosome has the error affects different things in the baby's body. Some of the babies with damage in the teen chromosome numbers do not live, or not for long, because it affects more serious areas in the body. Our little girl lived only two years, and she was sick the whole time that she lived."

"That's sad." I groped for words that would sound right. "I bet it was hard for you to lose her."

"Yes, it was." Her voice reflected a sense of loss. "However, it doesn't seem to affect babies as much when the chromosome damage is in the twenties."

I watched her as she shuffled through the papers on her clipboard until she found a small booklet.

"Here's a little book that I think will help you. Your baby will not learn things naturally as a normal baby does, and she will have to be taught how to do everything by stimulation. This book was written by the mother of a mentally retarded child and outlines ways to work with retarded children."[1] (A bibliography of books that have helped us will be listed at the end of this book.)

The social worker was the first person to give me an idea of what Lorie would be like. Somehow knowing what lay ahead was reassuring.

"Hi, honey," my husband greeted me, as he came strolling through the doorway.

"What are you doing here? Don't you have to work?" I asked.

"When I told my bosses about Lorie, they told me to come here and be with you. They told me to take the rest of the week off."

"Really? Will you still get paid?" His news had surprised me.

"Yes," Don answered as he leaned over to give me a quick kiss. "They all felt you needed me, and to tell you the truth, I wouldn't have been able to do a good job at work."

"I'm glad; I do need you. I can hardly believe they are being so nice to us."

"Me neither. I was shocked when they told me. I didn't waste any time getting over here so I could be with the two of you."

How thankful I was to Don's bosses for being so understanding. Things seemed so much better with my husband here.

"Why don't you get a paper gown so you can hold her?" I knew how anxious Don was to hold Lorie.

He didn't even answer me; he just hurried out of the room and down the hall to find a nurse. He came back so quickly that I hardly knew he was gone. He put on the gown, and I handed Lorie to him.

She was so small she practically fit in the palm of his hand. She moved a bit but quickly settled down and went right back to sleep.

I was so happy to be with Don. Together we could adjust to our special daughter before we took her home.

We talked a lot in the next few hours about how we felt, our fears, how we would do everything possible to help our daughter. We didn't have much hope—everything looked bleak and black to us then. The only thing we knew for sure was that we were going to take her home and learn everything we could to help her!

Later that day, a lady stopped outside the entrance to my room and checked her clipboard before entering.

"Cobbs?" she addressed us in an impersonal tone.

"Yes?" Don answered.

She introduced herself as a pediatrics doctor and told us it had been her colleague who had talked to me the day before.

"My colleague," she started out bluntly, "told you that your daughter is Mongoloid, and I'm here to tell you that I am making arrangements for your daughter's karyotype test to be done. I will order the test, and they should have it completed before you leave the hospital. The results will be back in three to four weeks. The test will tell us not only if she is Mongoloid for sure but also what type she is. Most Mongoloid babies are Trisomy 21. This means it was a result of a mistake in cell division causing the blueprint to go off in the beginning. If this is the kind she is, it means it shouldn't happen again if you decide to have another baby."

"You mean there are different types?" Don inquired.

"Yes, there are three main ones, and one is hereditary." She paused for a minute before she continued.

"Have you decided if you would like to give up your baby?"

"What?" Don said. This was one option we hadn't considered at all.

"You do not have to keep your baby. You can sign papers today to give her over to the state. If you sign them, you don't even have to go home with her. They will put her in an institution and take care of her so you don't have to be bothered."

You're making me mad! Where do you come from to believe you just get rid of babies when they aren't born perfect? Why do you even think we want to give her up?

"No, we are keeping her," Don answered.

"You know, if you keep her, you are in for a lot of problems and hard years ahead. She will be a lot of work, and she will not be able to do much of anything. It will be especially hard when you have to teach her about her monthly period."

Who cares about that now! We'll cross that bridge when the time comes!

"It's your decision," she continued, "but if you take her home and change your mind, you can still turn her over to the state. You can do it whenever you want to, even if you have had her home for a few years."

I can't believe people really believe this way. Why do they want to punish a baby for not being born perfect?

I was stunned! Had this really taken place? Did she actually believe this way?

"Oh, Don," I wailed, "is our baby going to be a vegetable?" That doctor did not say one positive thing to us! In my mind I could see Lorie not ever doing much of anything and being hard to care for. I did not remember the other things I had been told before the doctor's visit.

In those first moments after she left, and throughout

the next day, we had very little hope. We even questioned if we were making the right decision to take her home.

"Maybe we shouldn't have had another baby," Don said dejectedly.

"Why?" I asked. "I don't understand why you are saying that." *Did he blame himself?*

"You know the doctor told us that my sperm isn't very good. Maybe that's the reason she's Mongoloid."

"Oh, Don, don't blame yourself. It just happened. Maybe it was something I did during the time I was expecting her." I hadn't told Don before, but I had been worried that I had done something, too.

The obstetrician was our next visitor, and he couldn't have arrived at a better time.

"I've just examined your baby, and she has newborn jaundice," he told us.

"Oh, no! What else can go wrong today?" I was nearly in tears. "Why did this have to happen to her?"

"Newborn jaundice is common in new babies. In fact, one-third of all normal newborns develop some jaundice on the third or fourth day of life," the doctor explained to me. "This is especially true with newborns who are small in size."

"All babies," he continued, "are born with a high red blood count. As this red blood count becomes normal, the extra red blood cells are destroyed and form bilirubin in the baby's blood. The baby's liver usually removes the bilirubin from the body. If the bilirubin level in the body becomes too high, it could be harmful to the baby."

"Is it serious?" I asked him.

"No, so you don't have to be overly concerned with it. We will put Lorie under a special lamp to bring down her bilirubin count. You will not be able to have your baby very much, as she needs to stay under the bilirubin light as much as possible; the nurses will bring your baby to you for feeding time.''

''Is it like yellow jaundice?'' Don asked.

''No, and it is *not* contagious. When your baby's newborn jaundice disappears, it will not recur,'' the doctor answered.

''Do you know how long it will take for her bilirubin count to come down?'' I asked.

''No, but I hope it will be down so you can take her home with you.''

With the newborn jaundice talk out of the way, Don told him the events that had transpired since we had last seen him.

''I was going to tell you,'' he said to me. ''I'm sorry about the way it was handled.'' I felt better knowing that he hadn't wanted it to happen that way.

I nervously rubbed my hands together trying to gather up enough courage to ask the doctor a question. Finally, my desire for the answer was stronger than my fear of what the answer might be, and I asked him, ''Was it something I did while I was carrying her?''

''No, don't blame yourself. It happened in the beginning stages of development when the twenty-first chromosome failed to divide correctly, causing an abnormal reproductive cell. This resulted in your baby being born Mongoloid. You had no control over this.''

After the doctor had gone, we walked to the nursery to see how our baby was getting along in her treatment. She was protesting with intermittent cries, while furiously thrashing her arms and legs around. There was no doubt she didn't like this at all!

As I watched her through the nursery window, questions were running across my mind: *Is it normal to feel guilty as I have? Do parents of other handicapped babies feel this way, too?* I had so many questions, but no answers.

"Don," I said with deep sadness, "what else can go wrong!"

"Nothing, I hope," he answered.

We had a favorite nurse, one who was kind and helpful to us. She followed us into my room as we returned from the nursery.

Don asked her, "Do you think we could get some help that's positive? We would like to meet someone who has a Mongoloid child. They would really know what's up, since they have been through it."

"I'll go to the front desk and get the Retarded Association's number. You can call them and see what they can do for you."

When she returned, Don dialed their number and set up an appointment for the next evening. I could hardly wait for them to come—there was so much we needed to know. And they would understand; they had been through this!

There was no doubt we needed someone to give us some hope. Would this nightmare ever get any better? How much more could we take?

A Ray of Hope

A friend loves at all times (Prov. 17:17).

The arrival of Thursday morning found me watching Jan get ready to go home. She was excited, because for the first time out of three sons' births she was able to take her new son home with her from the hosptial. The first two babies had had to remain hospitalized because of newborn jaundice.

When her husband arrived with the clothes to take their new son home in, I asked her if I could see what a size zero looked like next to Lorie. I was anxious to see if a size zero would fit.

"Sure," Jan answered as she brought over the tiny sleeper. I put it next to Lorie—it was too large! If I were to put it on Lorie, she would swim in it!

Don happened to walk into the room while I was putting the small sleeper up to Lorie's small body.

"Don, a size zero will not fit her at all! What are we going to do?"

Don laughed, "I guess I'm going shopping for doll clothes. An eighteen-inch size should fit her."

The nurse arrived to dress Jan and Gene's little son,

and soon we were saying good-bye and promising to call each other soon.

The rest of the day passed quickly with the normal routines in a hospital's daily schedule and with friends coming to visit me. Their coming reassured me that people weren't going to desert us because Lorie wasn't born normal. Don went shopping in the afternoon and found out that trying to find a doll's outfit the day after Christmas takes special skill. He did not find one and had to try again later in the week.

The Parent Advocate couple arrived shortly after seven o'clock, and introduced themselves as Pat and Mary. We shared our sad story, our fears, and our feelings of hopelessness.

Mary, in the chair beside me, said, "The first thing we learned is not to believe all that the doctors say. They aren't always right. Our Sandy has proved her doctors wrong a great many times, as have other Down's children we know."

"The pediatrics doctor had us believing Lorie wasn't going to do much of anything," I said.

"That's not true," she answered me. "Your baby will do things like normal babies, only at a slower rate. Normal babies learn naturally, but Down's babies have to be taught how to do things. Down's children, who used to not walk until the age of four or five, are now walking around the age of two, if they have been taught. The point I'm trying to get across is that Down's children are doing almost everything a lot earlier with this extra help."

"How will I know what to do to help her?"

"Our county is trying to start an Infant Stimulation Program in which the public health nurse teaches you exercises and things to do with Lorie to help her get a good start. When Lorie is two, she can go to the D.A.C., where she will get even more help."

"What's that?" Don asked before I could get the same words out.

"The Day Activity Center. It's a special school for the preschool handicapped child. Mentally retarded children of different types are helped to learn more things. Here, in addition to teachers, the school has speech and physical therapists. The earlier the teachers start working with these kids, the better the kids learn and are able to get along the rest of their lives. When our Sandy was little, four was the youngest the child could be to go to D.A.C. Now the age is two."

Whew! Sending a two-year-old to school was something to think about!

"What will it be like taking care of Lorie?"

"Much like any other baby. Basically, love her and take care of her like any other baby."

Mary, who worked at one of the D.A.C.'s, was so enthusiastic about her work there: "I get so excited and thrilled whenever I see one of these little children make progress—it's a rewarding job."

She's giving us the first real ray of hope that we have had in days. She's a positive person. Maybe there is a future for our little girl!

"Why did the doctor give us the impression she would be like a vegetable?" I asked.

Mary answered, "Most of the doctors do not know very much about mental retardation and learn about it only for a short time in medical school. We have a Parent Panel that goes to hospitals and doctors' groups telling them what it's like. Our Parent Panel came to this hospital and talked to the staff this fall."

When Pat and Mary left, we had set up a tentative appointment to get together so that I could meet Sandy. I did want to see what an older Down's Syndrome child was like.

Pat and Mary had been such a help to us, and for the

first time since we learned the sad news, we had hope! We knew we had not made a wrong decision in keeping her, and we knew that there was help for us to manage with her at home.

Don and I parted that evening with our first real ray of hope—a tiny straw to grasp at, but at least somewhere to start.

(Later I was to learn in a booklet why the term Down's Syndrome is preferable to Mongoloid. It stated, "Dr. Langdon Down first described this syndrome about one hundred years ago, and it came to bear his name— Down's Syndrome. Because of a vague resemblance in the face of such a child to the Asian races, he was described as a 'mongol,' and hence, the old terms 'mongolism' and 'mongoloid.' However, it is incorrect to associate the condition with Asians, who are indeed offended by the term. It is considered demeaning and developmentally inappropriate to refer to a child as a 'Mongoloid' "[2])

After Don left that evening I met another mother at the nursery, and the conversation changed to Lorie's handicap.

"What's wrong with your little girl? I heard some of the ladies say one of the newborn babies was handicapped, but I didn't know which one."

"She has Down's Syndrome." I answered, and went on to tell her a little more about it.

"I'm sorry—that must be hard for you. The same day that I heard about your baby, some of the other mothers were talking about a mother who had had a baby of a different sex from what she wanted. She refused to see the baby, hold it, or feed it."

"How can she act that way?" I asked. "If I were to meet her, I would tell her to get down on her knees and thank God that her baby was normal. Some people don't know when they're well off, do they?"

"No, I guess not," she answered.

Shortly afterward I went back to my room, still thinking about the mother who didn't want her baby. I could hardly believe someone would act that way.

The next morning my new acquaintance came by as she was leaving and gave me two of her flower arrangements. "I have so very many," she told me, "and I would like you and your little girl to have a couple of them." Her kindness really touched my heart and reassured me there were nice people in the world—people who give from their hearts.

Friday, my last full day in the hospital, my parents arrived just before the end of hospital visiting hours. They had traveled several hours to get there and stopped to see me before going to our home. The hospital bent the rule and told them they could stay past the end of visiting hours.

"Something is wrong with our baby," I told them after the small talk had taken place.

"We thought so," my mom said. "Don didn't say anything on the phone, but it was just the way his voice sounded."

We took them down to the nursery to see her. She looked so tiny clad only in a diaper, giving us a good look at her small legs and arms.

"She doesn't like being under the light, does she?" Dad said as he watched her angrily crying, kicking, and screaming.

"No," Don answered him. "She hasn't liked it from the first moment they put her there."

"Maybe the doctors are wrong in their diagnosis, and she is really all right." I could tell Mom really wanted Lorie to be normal; by now, I was starting to accept the fact that she probably was not.

"Poor little one," Dad said, "to have to start out her life handicapped. She sure is a cutie. I can hardly wait to hold her." Dad has a way, in times of misfortune, of bouncing back right away. He was showing us that somehow we could start again with Lorie and revise our original dream.

After they left, I lay trying to sleep and thinking of all that had happened during the last few days. Our lives had surely changed and would never be the same. I fell asleep with the hope that I would be taking our baby home the next morning.

With the arrival of a new day, I anxiously awaited the news of whether Lorie was coming home with me, and I was elated when the nurse told me, "Her bilirubin count is way down and her birth weight is four pounds fifteen ounces, and since it is so close to five pounds, the doctor is going to release her."

Thank heaven! I get to take her home!

Mom arrived carrying two large brown bags. "The men folk will be up in a minute. They're parking the car."

"Did you find some clothes for Lorie to wear home?"

"Yes, but Don had to go to quite a few stores. He finally found this little dress." She took out a small, green satin dress. It was cute, and I thought our baby would look darling in it.

"I bought a doll so that we could get more clothes from it." She undressed the doll, giving me its hat, coat, and tights.

How many other moms take their babies home in doll clothes? I could hardly wait for the nurse to come and dress our little princess.

After the doctor checked us, he signed our release, and the nurse came to dress our baby. She slipped the tiny clothing on Lorie, and we all admired the baby. The nurse showed her off to some of the other staff before wrapping her in her blankets. We were off, leaving the hospital, and heading home.

Oh, Lorie, I thought during the ride home. *I hope I will be the right mother for you, since you have arrived needing a lot more care than a normal baby.* I looked at Lorie wrapped in a pink blanket, and I thought, *Here's your home and the start of your life here.* Don opened the door and we went inside to begin our life with the newest member of our family.

Love Tested

Every good thing bestowed and every perfect gift is from above, coming down from the Father of lights, with whom there is no variation, or shifting shadow (James 1:17).

Lorie had just finished drinking the amount of milk she wanted and was looking around at me and the things that she could see. I leaned back in the rocking chair and moved back and forth gently. She liked the rocking and settled down and fell asleep. We had managed to make it through the first month, though it had been quite a month!

My mind drifted back to the Saturday morning we had brought her home. When I had stepped through the doorway, I handed Lorie to Don and knelt and opened my arms wide for Kevin. He came running toward me, obviously happy that his mom was home again. Don unwrapped Lorie's blankets and knelt, enabling the three small boys (two were my nephews) to get a good view of her.

"She sure is small!" Darren, the oldest of the three boys, commented.

"Was I ever that small?" Paul asked his mommy.

"Yes, you were small, but not quite as small as little Lorie is," Peg told him.

Don stood and handed Lorie to me. "That's enough, boys; the baby has to go to bed."

"Go to bed! She just got home!" Kevin said with surprise.

"Yes, newborn babies sleep a lot of the time. Someday, when she gets older, she won't sleep so much, and you will be able to play with her."

Thus began the first day at home. The days were noisy ones with a house full of people, three rambunctious boys, and a new baby whose crying let us know she was there. Besides the relatives being around, friends and neighbors stopped to see Lorie and drop off gifts. It was reassuring to me to have them come to visit.

On one of our first days at home, Mom and my sister went downtown to shop, and returned with a large piece of aqua material that Mom had found on a remnant table.

"I thought this would be nice material for me to make Lorie some small nightgowns," Mom said. There was no doubt Lorie needed something to wear; nothing fit her except the doll clothes we had bought.

Mom took a doll nightgown, drafted a pattern from it, and made three small gowns. These would be Lorie's main wardrobe for her first month of life.

I was ingenious with the rest of her clothing articles. I cut Pampers in half, and then they fit perfectly. Lorie's booties were tiny ones that a girl friend of mine had found. The tiny T-shirts swam on her, but by pulling them together tighter and pinning them, they fit. It certainly was interesting having such a small baby!

One day, shortly before my parents were to go home, the phone rang. I put Lorie on the couch and went into

39

the kitchen to answer it. "Mrs. Cobb," a female voice addressed me, "this is the lab at the hospital. The karyotype test that was done on your baby before she left didn't take, and we were wondering if you could bring her down for another one."

"When do you want me to bring her in?"

"How about ten o'clock tomorrow morning?"

"That's okay," I answered.

The next morning, with my dad at the wheel of the car, we drove the short distance for our lab appointment. I was sitting in the front with Lorie on my lap and looking out the window at the snow-covered banks. The roads were slippery, and I was glad Dad was driving. Mom was in the back seat with Kevin and my sister's oldest boy, Darren.

My feelings during the ride were those of apprehension, concern, and sorrow. I was somewhat uptight wondering how Lorie would react to being poked with a needle again.

When we arrived at the hospital, Mom, Lorie, and I went immediately to the lab. As we waited, I couldn't help but remember a few days earlier when I had been waiting for the doctor to come to the mothers' lounge. Somehow, this time of waiting wasn't as hard as that one had been.

A lady came to get Lorie and they disappeared from view. Shortly after, we could hear Lorie scream, and it bothered me. She had been poked with needles so much during her hospital stay that I really hated to have her hurt again.

The lady returned with Lorie; it certainly hadn't taken long. "She sure is a small one," she said as she handed my baby back to me. "We had a time finding a vein on her with everything being so small!"

I wrapped her back up in her blankets and was happy to see she was no longer fussing. *I hope this one takes*, I thought as we left the hospital and drove back home.

My wish did not come true. Just before my folks' visit was over, the lab called again.

"I'm sorry, but that blood test didn't take either. This time, would you just take her to the Children's Hospital lab?"

I was not the least bit happy that Lorie had to have the test again. How much more would she have to go through? Would this nightmare ever end?

Since they scheduled this test for after my parents' visit, Don took the morning off from work to take us to the lab. It was another cold, winter day, and our view was again snow-covered banks. Trees, whose lovely summer array had been shed in the fall, stood with straight, bare branches with bits of snow clinging to them. Some hardy people were out in the frigid weather, bundled up to endure it.

We entered the hospital, and then got off the elevator in front of some nursery windows. The sign to the lab area pointed to the left, and we headed in that direction. We soon joined several other parents and their children in waiting.

Before long a young woman called Lorie's name, and we followed her into a small examining room. There, a man with a white lab coat gave the young woman instructions on what he wanted done for the lab test. I watched as she lined up the equipment: needle, test tube, etc.

"We will let you hold, love, and comfort your baby while we draw the blood," she cheerfully told me. I held my tiny baby and turned my head away—I didn't want to watch. Lorie protested loudly. *My poor baby*, I thought. *How much you are having to go through! I hope this is the end!*

"That's it," the lab technician told me. I turned my head back to see my baby who was still crying.

Lorie

"I'm finished hurting you with the needle," the young woman soothed Lorie. "Now your mommy can hold and love you so you can forget this awful hurt." I picked Lorie up and cuddled her; with my comforting her, she quit crying. I was relieved this was over with!

This had to be it! If it wasn't, I would scream!

During our drive back home, I secretly hoped that this test would prove she wasn't Down's. I think deep down I really knew she was, but I still held onto a small amount of hope that maybe, just maybe, she wasn't. How much easier things would be if she weren't Down's and was a normal little girl instead.

Lorie was an easy baby to take care of—she cried only when she had a definite need. And her cry was not very loud compared to her brother's piercing cry.

It wasn't easy getting used to her nasal breathing though; she really sounded awful. In fact, it sounded worse than it was. "The reason her breathing sounds so funny," the doctor had told us, "is that her nasal passages are so much smaller than a normal baby's. You don't have to be overly concerned with it. I must tell you, though, that she will be more susceptible to pneumonia, bronchitis and any other upper respiratory ailment." To help Lorie breathe, I laid her with her head elevated on a small pillow.

I started reading books and pamphlets trying to learn as much as I could about Down's Syndrome. I learned that one in four Down's children have bad hearts, and that it would usually show up before the age of four months. Another book explained all the various birth defects and what causes them. I learned that we could have had a baby with a handicap much worse than Lorie's.

Oddly enough, one pamphlet I had sent for from the National Retarded Association had a section in it that would save Lorie's life. The pamphlet arrived in the morning mail on the day the incident happened. That night Don had left to go back to work. Kevin and I were still at the supper table eating our dessert when I heard Lorie whimper, as she did from time to time. I usually didn't get concerned unless she let out a demanding cry. But for some reason, without any conscious thought on my part, I went to her. I picked her up from the small porta-crib and was startled to see she wasn't breathing! Panic engulfed my whole body!

Oh, God—What am I going to do? Oh, why did this have to happen when Don isn't here? I was scared. I dashed out into the living room with her, trying to decide what to do.

Kevin had just let Marie in and I was relieved to see her!

"Marie!" I screamed. "My baby's not breathing, and I don't know what to do!" Poor Marie! She had a way of always arriving in my crisis times!

Then I remembered the section in the pamphlet that I had read that afternoon on how to help your child's breathing if he has a lot of nasal discharge. Maybe she had sucked some milk or phlegm back into her lungs. I quickly gave Marie the baby and got the book.

"Sit in the chair and do what I read to you!"

Marie, who was as scared as I was, sat in the chair and did exactly what I read. "Put her face down in your lap with her head hanging over the end of your legs. Start pushing with your hands on her back from the lower back to the shoulders."

As Marie was doing what I had instructed, I ran into the kitchen to call Don. I reached him about a minute before the news was to go on the air, and it was a good thing, for after the cable news program started, they would not answer the phone for the next half hour. Terry, the young camera woman, answered the phone. She didn't want to let me talk to Don, since it was so near air time, until she heard my panic-stricken voice say, "It's an emergency!" She flung the phone at Don, and he caught the receiver. "Don, our baby isn't breathing!"

"I will be right home!" I heard him slam the receiver onto the phone.

Marie had been doing what I had instructed her to do for only a short time when some phlegm came out, and Lorie started breathing again and, with that, crying. *Thank God she is all right!* I breathed a sigh of relief, and tears rolled down my cheeks. I picked up my little daughter and cuddled her tightly.

Don came running in the door shortly afterward. He had rushed the nine-mile stretch home having to stop only for one red light, and was thankful a cop didn't stop him for going too fast! We hadn't lost Lorie, and I, though relieved, was still nervous and upset. It had been quite an ordeal!

Don put his arm around me, and we both gazed at our tiny daughter who was now calm and quiet.

"I was really scared!" Don said. "I don't think I have ever been that scared in my life. I didn't want to lose our daughter."

"I know. I didn't want to lose her either. Thank heaven that booklet arrived today; the information in it saved her life!"

There was no doubt we loved our little baby. The fear of losing her had really scared us and made us realize that whether or not she was perfect wasn't important—we wanted her as she was. She was our daughter!

Don called the emergency ward at the hospital and was told there was not much to do now—just to keep an eye on her for a couple of days and to bring her in right away if her lips or fingernails started turning blue.

Don went to the basement and brought up our

laundry basket, and we made a little bed for her in that. This way I could keep her by my side and check her often. I wanted to be sure she was okay.

Depression had been my constant companion ever since the doctor told me the sad news. I cried a lot. I felt as if a black rain cloud hung over me constantly, and my outlook concerning life was bleak. I was full of self-pity and worried about Lorie's future. I saw very little good that could come out of this situation. There was no doubt I had been zapped with a problem I didn't know how to handle myself.

One night I asked Don if the kids and I could go to Rochester for a visit; I felt that a change of scenery and seeing some of my friends might keep my mind off feeling sorry for us and for our baby. We had lived in Rochester for five years and had several friends there. Don agreed; he knew he had an outlet to take his mind off of Lorie—his job offered a diversion. I, on the other hand, remained with Lorie day and night with little opportunity to think of anything else. I know you can't run away from your problems, but Don too thought a week away with something different to think about could be beneficial.

Our friends received the children and me warmly. Lorie was greeted into the world just like any other baby.

I took Lorie to the place where I had worked in Rochester. I showed her off, and the girls admired her and commented on how small she was. I didn't tell them about Lorie's handicap this visit; we were starting to tell a few people at a time, but it was a slow process. It got easier as time went on, and we found out we were not receiving negative reactions.

One morning during my visit I called a girl friend and asked if we could come for a visit.

Lorie

"I'd love to see you!" Amy exclaimed. "We haven't seen each other for ages."

I bundled up the children and myself, and we drove across town to see Amy. She saw us drive up and rushed out to meet us. I had told her about Lorie on the phone, and she greeted me with a hug. "I'm sorry, Mary Ann," she said simply.

When we were settled in the kitchen, she poured us each a cup of hot tea.

"I was really sorry to hear about your losing your boys last year," I said. Amy had had a rough year; her first son was born seven weeks early, lived a week, and died. She had gotten pregnant again almost right away, and the second boy also arrived seven weeks early, stillborn. "How did you manage to get through it?"

"The first time I decided anyone could have some bad luck, but the second time, I was angry and bitter. It took me an awfully long time to get over it."

I couldn't imagine losing two babies in one year—in fact, I couldn't imagine losing one. I felt such deep sadness for her. "You have had things worse than I," I said.

"I think you have it worse." She picked up the plate of cookies and held them toward me. "Have one?"

I took a cookie and answered, "How can you say that? Your babies are dead—I still have mine."

"Yes, but you still have your problem. My problems have gone away, and time is healing the hurt. It was terrible at the time, but it's getting better."

The phone rang, taking Amy away and giving me time to think about what she had just told me. Hadn't she gone through something worse? Sure, it was getting better for her, but we still had our baby. I looked at Lorie and saw that she was asleep. She looked so cute.

When Amy returned, she told me, "Let me try to explain it better. It was rough for me when I lost two sons in one year. It was the worst thing that had ever happened to me. As time passed, I understood that life continues.''

The afternoon passed quickly as we talked about Amy's new pregnancy and more about Lorie and her handicap. I was glad I had gone to visit her. She had helped me see that people can adjust to misfortunes. I was sure, in time, our hurts would heal, and we too would be adjusted to it.

My mini-vacation to Rochester was good for me, and I was ready to get back to the everyday routine.

After coming home I kept thinking about Amy. Why had she lost two babies? Why did some people have six, seven, or eight perfectly healthy babies while others have lost babies or have handicapped ones? Could I cope if I had lost two babies? Were my problems worse than hers?

They say children are a gift from God. If that's so, I wondered, why had He taken Amy's two sons and given us an imperfect baby?

Would there ever be answers for my endless questions?

I Need Jesus

If you confess with your mouth Jesus as Lord, and
believe in your heart that God raised Him from the dead,
you shall be saved; for with the heart man believes,
resulting in righteousness, and with the mouth he con-
fesses, resulting in salvation (Rom. 10:9,10).

Not too long after our Rochester visit, Lorie and I
braved the cold January weather and drove to the
clinic. Lorie was going for her check-up. She was five
weeks old.

At the clinic we followed a nurse into a small examining room where she asked me to undress Lorie down to
her diaper. I was anxious to see how much Lorie
weighed now. Her first check-up at two weeks had put
her at five pounds, nine-and-a-half ounces, and she
had stayed at her birth length of eighteen inches.

The nurse returned, picked up Lorie, and put her on
the scale. Lorie squirmed and protested. "Hmm . . .
seven pounds even." She wrote Lorie's weight on
Lorie's chart and in the small book they had given me.
"That's a good increase. Now, lay her on the paper on
the examining table, and I'll measure her."

I watched the nurse mark the paper at the top of Lorie's head and the bottom of her feet. She measured the length between the two marks: "She has grown two inches. She is now twenty inches."

We then waited awhile for the doctor. Since our regular doctor was gone for the day, I had chosen to see the doctor who had delivered Lorie. He was surprised to see us when he walked through the door. "Hi . . . how's the baby?"

"So far, so good. She is an easy baby to take care of," I responded.

"Good. Let's check her and see how she is doing health-wise. Would you put her on the examining table?"

I waited apprehensively as the doctor checked her. Would he find something this time? Would he find a bad heart? I worried a lot about her physical health, because she had more chances than a normal baby of having something wrong.

"She's checking out okay. I don't see any problem areas. Let's take her blood count to see how that is. I'll have the nurse come in and do it."

I breathed a sigh of relief. "Do you know if the results have come back from Lorie's chromosome tests?" I asked. "They haven't called and told us anything yet."

The nurse came in, and Lorie protested the prick of the pin. After the nurse left, the room seemed strangely quiet. I was nervous—part of me wanted to know; the other part of me wanted to wait longer. As long as I didn't know the results, I could hold onto a small amount of hope that maybe, just maybe, the doctors were wrong and Lorie was normal.

"Yes, they are back. I will have to read them before I can explain them to you. Oh, the blood test is done and her blood count is a little low, but nothing to be concerned about." I watched him sit at the small desk and look over the papers.

I was uptight. I fiddled with my hands and moved nervously on the hard chair where I was sitting. *Do I really want to know the results? Oh, hurry! I can't stand the suspense!*

The doctor put the papers down and looked at me. I held my breath. "Yes, she is Down's Syndrome. She is Trisomy 21, just as I suspected after I delivered her. This is the freak one where something goes wrong in the beginning stages of development; it is not the hereditary one. You should not have another Down's if you decide to have more babies, but your chances will be somewhat higher because you have had one."

The words sunk in. In one way, the results didn't surprise me, and in other ways, I was disappointed. How much easier things would be if she were normal!

One cold, snowy January morning, Mary, from the ARC parent advocate program, and her three daughters came to see us. Sandy, the Down's Syndrome child, was the middle child. Sandy was small, about the size of Kevin. She really didn't look any different from any other little girl her size. She and Kevin hit it right off, and away they went to play.

Mary held Lorie, "I just love to hold babies," she told me.

Sandy rushed in to show her mother a toy she liked. She saw the baby, and her face lit with excitement. Pointing at the baby, she mumbled some words I couldn't understand. "Sandy," her mother addressed her, "what do you think of the baby? Do you like her?"

Sandy nodded her head affirmatively and patted the baby gently.

Sandy certainly isn't a passive child. She is an active

little girl, only slower in development. Lorie will be able to do things, too, when she is older.

It made me feel good to see Sandy and to know that Lorie would be able to do things, too. "What will Lorie's speech be like?" Sandy was the first Down's child I had seen, besides Lorie, and Sandy's speech was limited because she had a cleft lip and palate.

"She could have good speech; several children at the D.A.C. talk very well and very plainly."

"Weren't you afraid of having another handicapped baby when you were carrying Shelly?"

"Shelly came fifteen months after Sandy, and I was more concerned for Sandy's cleft lip and palate than I was about the Down's. We were thankful when Shelly arrived okay."

"Was it hard having them close in age with Sandy being handicapped?"

"It turned out to be nice, though a lot of work. Shelly became Sandy's own Infant Stimulation Program, as Sandy learned a lot of things from watching Shelly. I even potty-trained them together."

"How did people feel about your keeping her?" I asked.

"The doctors advised us to give her up. When Sandy was sixteen months old and in the hospital with pneumonia, even our minister thought I was foolish to have kept her and for spending my time in the hospital with her. He thought I should go home to my normal girls."

"Nine years later, the doctors are still advising people to give up their babies. Times haven't changed much!" I exclaimed.

Mary was so helpful that afternoon, as she answered my many questions—believe me, I had a lot of them! I was glad I had gotten to know her right away, and I knew I now had a nice, new friend.

Lorie

With the passing of time, and knowing Lorie was indeed Down's, I found my adjusting getting much better. The first days I had been in a deep depression, and I made it through those days hour by hour. I progressed to making it day by day. Now I found myself going several days without depression. I was returning to normal and beginning to adjust to this situation.

I found that as I was coping more I was shifting to another area. I wanted to learn all I could about Down's.

It's funny how one thing leads to another, but my jumbled thoughts and many, many unanswered questions led me into the most searching period of my life. My questions led to other areas, not just those concerning "Why?" or even "Why us?" I had always been a moderately curious person, but now I seemed frantic to have some answers to these questions.

At this time, I did not know that my curiosity and searching would bring another change in our lives: a good change that would lead us in another direction.

My searching for answers started with some books that the local Retarded Association lent me, and I was able to start learning more about Down's Syndrome. I spent days reading as much as I could. Not only did I learn a lot, but it helped calm some of my fears of the unknown.

It's funny; a few months earlier, I had never given a handicapped child a thought, but Lorie's birth was changing my world. *How much we take a normal birth for granted!* We sure had with Kevin, and though we were excited about his new accomplishments, we didn't realize how great it was that he could do things on his own.

I also started facing my feelings. How did I really feel about this? At first I had been hurt, angry, and disappointed. My fears about Lorie's health caused me to be apprehensive. I worried if I was the right mother for her. It was scary realizing all that would be involved in rearing a special child.

Now I found that though I was still hurt, my beginning to accept her being a Down's baby was causing a lot of my fears to go away. The more I learned about Down's Syndrome, the more it helped me to accept it. It was grinding out my fears of the unknown. I was, at long last, ready to meet the future and was developing some positive feelings. With help for Lorie, why couldn't she be and do the best that is possible? I was determined to give her the chance, and was sure it could be done.

Curiosity has a way at times of leading people into strange subjects. It did for me one afternoon when I sat down to take a break from my household chores. I turned on the television to find Mike Douglas interviewing two men on the subject of reincarnation. The whole subject sounded strange to me, and I could hardly believe that people really believed this! Long after the program was over, I found myself thinking about what had been said.

In fact, that evening we were to entertain a girl who was interested in this subject. She told of things she had read, such as coming back as someone else, having a third eye in the middle of your forehead, and about being able to float out of your body at night.

I passed off her remarks because I thought the whole thing sounded a bit strange. I could hardly believe it. I certainly wasn't going to read any of the books she mentioned to see if she were telling the truth!

When Don and I went to bed that evening, the subject was still on my mind. I suddenly became afraid. I didn't want to float out of my body; I didn't want to think that after I died I would keep coming back! The night darkness has a way of making fears worse, and tonight my fears were grasping me. I clung to Don as tightly as I could and became angry when he turned his back to me. *This is silly to be afraid of the things she had told me.* I tried to reason with myself, but the fears hung on, and I got little sleep that night.

I must have fallen asleep in the wee hours of the morning, and I awoke with the same subject on my mind. I lay in bed letting the thoughts run wild. A booming voice seemed to cross my mind saying, "Oh, Mary Ann, you know this is ridiculous!"

If that's so, I thought, *what really is the truth.* I got out of bed to begin my day's activities and then forgot the whole incident.

The subject came up again three weeks later. We happened to be driving by a new shopping mall when Don asked me if I would like to go in.

"Yes, I'm curious to see what a mall built on three levels looks like. Can we go to a bookstore when we get inside?" I didn't know why I wanted to go there.

"All right." He gave me a funny look. I'm sure that with all the stores to visit, he was surprised I wanted to go to a bookstore.

We found one on the top level. As soon as I entered, I was drawn to the religious book section. I rarely looked for books in this section. Thoughts about reincarnation filled my mind again; I looked to see if there was a book that would tell the truth about it.

Scanning the book titles, I stopped at Hal Lindsey's book *Satan Is Alive and Well on the Planet Earth.* I picked up the book and glanced through the pages.

"Don, there's something in this book that might answer some of my questions about reincarnation; he talks about the occult."

"Get it if you want to." Don was agreeable.

Next to this book was another of Lindsey's books,

The Late Great Planet Earth, which told about the end times. It looked interesting to me.

"Can I get this one, too?"

"Okay, give me the books, and I'll go pay for them."

On the way home I started reading the Satan book. "This book is really interesting," I told Don.

I did not know the Bible told such interesting things—I had never read much of the Bible. We went to a church that taught little from the Bible, and we just put in our time in church on Sunday.

On the night I finished the Satan book, I thought about Hal Lindsey's saying that to be in God's family you have to ask Jesus into your heart. I had never done that. I wanted to. I wanted to belong to God, to have Him help me and guide me, and I wanted to go to heaven. Jesus seemed to be saying, "I can carry the burden of your special baby." I wanted that, too.

"Dear Jesus," I said ever so softly, "please forgive my sins and come into my heart and be my Savior. I need and want You."

A calm peace came over me, and I felt good. I lay there a few minutes thinking over all I had learned in the last couple of days and of asking Jesus into my heart, until Don came into the bedroom to get ready for bed.

It would be ten months before I would really know what I had done. I became part of God's family, and in the interim, He led me by grace. I started changing; Jesus became real to me, and I found I could pray easily. Something definitely had happened to me!

Another Mother
Reaches Out

And we know that God causes all things to work together for good to those who love God, to those who are called according to His purpose (Rom. 8:28).

I called the public health nurse of our county to see if she could come out and see us. Mary had given us her name and number. The county was starting an Infant Stimulation Program through the public health nurse's office, and I wanted Lorie in it.

Lorie was about six weeks old when the short, dark-haired nurse came out to see us.

"We don't have much of a program set up yet," she said, "but we are starting on it. We have gone to the parents to offer help and give them some ideas to work with."

"When do you think it will be set up and organized?"

"I don't know for sure, but I hope it won't be too long. Do you have a blanket to lay on the floor? I'll run through a little test to see how Lorie is developing."

With the blanket on the floor, the nurse put Lorie on

it. She took a small book out of her bag and glanced through it. Then she held Lorie's hands and pulled her straight up. "Good!" she exclaimed. "She has good head control." I watched as she did various other small tests.

"Lorie's testing out normal right now. She hasn't started lagging yet. Most of the Down's babies are normal till about six months old, then they start falling behind in development."

She handed Lorie to me, and I sat on the couch with her.

"How are you doing?" the nurse asked me.

"Pretty good. It was hard at first, but it's getting better. Could you put me in touch with a mother of another Down's baby? I know a mother with an older child, but I would like to meet one with a baby."

"I'd like to give you someone's name, but I'm not supposed to give out private information. The person I'm thinking of could get angry. I will mention your name to her, and maybe she will call you."

I was disappointed. My friends with normal babies, though kind and sympathetic, didn't understand what I was going through. How I hoped there was a mother with a Down's baby who would want to meet me!

The phone rang one February afternoon. "Mary Ann," a female voice addressed me, "my name is Kathy, and I am the mother of a nine-month-old Down's boy."

I was excited! "I'm so glad you called me!"

"Your baby isn't very old, is she?" Kathy asked.

"No, she was born on Christmas Eve."

"Jeff was born June 30."

"A summer baby," I commented. "How were you told about it?"

"Our obstetrician had told John and me that we had a nice, healthy boy. We were happy; John had gone home; and I was resting when a strange doctor came into the room. He started talking about genes, chromosomes—I didn't know what he was talking about. Finally I asked him if our son was Mongoloid. He told me, 'That's exactly right!'

"It was a total shock, and I wanted John there. I had asked the doctor to talk to John on the phone and tell him what he had just told me," Kathy continued. "Instead, he walked around the bed, handed me the phone, and left! I was shocked and upset—John came right back to the hospital!"

"What did your obstetrician say?" I inquired.

"We had a good doctor. He told us not to believe Jeff was Down's until the blood test came back positive. Then he told us that our son needs us and to take him home and love him."

It surprised me that Don and I did not have a unique story, that someone else too had been told in an abrupt manner.

When I expressed my desire to meet them, Kathy invited us for a visit that evening.

We arrived about seven o'clock and met her and her husband, John, and their two sons, Johnny and Jeff. Johnny, about Kevin's age, and Kevin immediately headed for Johnny's room—they didn't care about the babies.

"Do you have any little cars?" Kevin's voice could be heard as they dashed into the bedroom.

Jeff was a small baby with thick, black hair. He grinned at us. She sat him on the floor.

"Don!" I exclaimed. "He's sitting up!" We knew that Lorie would do things later, but we thought it would be much later! Maybe she wouldn't be so far behind normal babies.

"Jeff isn't much behind normal babies, is he?"

"No, not so far," Kathy answered. "Your baby is

much smaller than I remember Jeff was, and I thought he was small. Jeff is enrolled in an Infant Stimulation Program in St. Paul, and we go once a week. Would you and Lorie like to go with us? We could trade off driving."

"What's it like?"

"It's a program where either a doctor or an assistant works with your baby, and a physical therapist shows you things to help in the physical areas."

"How did you get into this?"

"We found out about it when we lived in St. Paul. After we moved, the doctor, Dr. Lucille Poor, said we could continue in the program. It's quite a drive since we moved here, and it would be nice to have someone to go with."

Don and I agreed that it was a good idea.

"I'll talk to Dr. Poor and see if it is okay with her."

"I hope it works out for us to go. I would like Lorie to get the best possible start," I told her.

I was glad to meet Kathy and her husband, and we had a nice visit. I hoped Dr. Poor would say that it was okay—I really wanted to take Lorie to the Infant Stimulation Program.

A few days later Kathy called to tell me that Dr. Poor said it was okay for us to come. Kathy picked me up one Monday morning in March, and we made the half-hour drive to St. Paul-Ramsey County Mental Health Center.

Kathy parked in front of a three-story brick building. "This is it," she said. I followed her into the building, up to the third floor, and into a large empty room. On the left were long tables; in the front were mats spread on the floor; and to the right were chairs lined up against the wall. The room had a toy shelf, a nursery table, and a large, round table.

A red-haired lady came into the room carrying a large

coffee pot which she put on the round table and plugged in. She greeted us and then rushed over to the toy shelf and began taking toys down and putting them on the long tables.

We did not have to wait very long before other mothers started arriving. The room, which appeared large at first, seemed small as it started filling up. Kathy introduced me to the mothers and babies as they came in. I looked at each baby and marveled at the individuality of each one—each resembled his or her parent. For awhile there was mass confusion, with mothers and babies arriving, helpers setting up, and children crawling around and playing with the toys.

The two ladies, the red-haired one and a blonde one, were Dr. Poor's assistants. They helped work with the children by having them run through certain exercises listed on a sheet of paper. A volunteer arrived and she also worked with the children on these activities.

The three women would first look over the sheet of paper to see what they were to do and would then run through the items with the baby. The list included things like putting pegs in the holes, stacking blocks, and putting cubes through small holes. When the little ones did some of the things on their list, the ladies praised them.

The physical therapist arrived, and she took one of the children to a mat and began to work with him. I noticed that as she did each thing, she explained it to the mother so that she would know what to do at home.

Dr. Lucille Poor came into the room. She was older than I had thought she would be. Kathy introduced me to her. ''We want you to fill out some papers before you leave today, and I will work with your baby the very last thing.''

Dr. Poor had become interested in working with retarded children in earlier years when she had worked in state and general hospitals and saw how neglected these children were. "The physicians," she told me, "had done a great disservice by telling parents to forget their baby, that they would never want the baby, that they should face this fact right away. The parents were told that if they left the baby, the welfare department would arrange to put the baby in a foster home."

Much of the time, during the nine months that Lorie was in the program, Dr. Poor stressed to all of us that if a foster mother can take care of your baby, so can you! "The reason," she told us mothers, "is that going to a foster home is usually not the best thing for your baby. When he doesn't progress as he should, they send him off to another home. The child, sometimes by the age of seven months, has been in four or five homes and has not been able to make an attachment to any one person. Each time he is switched, he feels he has failed. And by the time he has been in four or five foster homes, he has a great fear of failure and will turn his face to the wall and will not eat."

Dr. Poor's program is for Down's infants up to the age of two years, when the child would usually go into a Day Activity Center. At the time she started her program, to her knowledge there were only eight other Infant Stimulation Programs in the country. Infant stimulation was in the early stages of development, and Lorie was getting in on the ground floor.

The physical therapist took Lorie to the mat; I followed and sat down on the floor. I was curious to see what she would do with a three-month-old. She took out a long round object and put a cloth over it while telling me that I could do the same thing with a rolling pin at home.

"This is to help with holding her head up." I watched as she placed Lorie on her stomach and put the round thing under Lorie's chest. During much of Lorie's physical therapy, she would cry and protest at the hard things (at least to her) she was made to do. "It isn't easy getting these little ones to do things, but you must, because these babies will not learn on their own," the physical therapist told me.

Dr. Poor came over toward the end of the morning session. "Would you like to put your baby on the nursery table and undress her to her diaper?"

Dr. Poor opened a drawer and got out the baby powder. "What I am going to teach you to do with your baby is a stimulation process. I would like you to do this with her every day."

I watched her put some baby powder on her hand and start to rub Lorie. "This stimulates the long and short muscles," she continued. "The purpose is to help the floppiness that many of these children have from poor muscle tone. The long muscles, like in the arms and legs, need to be stimulated, and particularly the lower back is weak and needs the stimulation.

"She seems to like it," I commented.

"Oh, yes. They love this. Many centers have suggested using an electric stimuli, but that is hard and cold, and I feel stimulation with the hands is far superior and gives the child the feeling of closeness and love. Human touch means a lot!"

She switched from rubbing Lorie's back, arms, legs, and stomach to rubbing her fingers and toes. "This is important not only for its motivation movements between the fingers and toes, but fingers are important for handling toys and other objects, dropping pellets into bottles, and things like that. Large muscles are important because of coordination. These youngsters have difficulties in walking and sitting up."

After the stimulation process was over and I had redressed Lorie, Dr. Poor gave me my first worksheet telling the things I was to do with Lorie at home.

"When she completes the tasks on this sheet, we will give you another sheet," she told me, handing me the one with the heading "Three Months Old."

She gave me another sheet which was geared for three to six months and had five different sections in it. "We also want you to keep a calendar. If Lorie does any of these things at home, or something new and different, write it in the blank spot for that day."

I left the center happy and determined that this would give Lorie a good start. After all, I had just seen other little ones there doing all kinds of things!

The next morning I started my assignment with giving Lorie her rub down. She liked it; there was no doubt about that!

I took out the sheets of paper and read them to see what I was supposed to be doing with her. The one headed "Three to Six Months" contained five pages. Each section contained a different area to work on, such as large muscle development, small muscle development, social/emotional development, cognitive (thinking) development, and language development.

The sheets told what normal infants could do at this age and explained how we could help our child to do these things. The sheets were broken down into what the infant could do, what you need to help (toys, other necessary articles), what needed to be done, and the reason for it.

The page that told about the small muscles showed how to strengthen those muscles and develop skill in the use of fingers and hands to manipulate objects. Each sheet, plus the three-months sheet, was giving me guides to help Lorie, and they didn't really involve that much work. These things would take a short amount of time each day.

One of the first things Dr. Poor was having me work with was an embroidery hoop with a ribbon attached to it. I learned that working with the hoop teaches eye and hand coordination. Moving the hoop over the baby from left to right tests the child's ability to follow it with his eyes and hands and indicates intelligence. This, though it couldn't reveal the amount of intelligence, could show one isolated incident of it.

Dr. Poor had us ring a bell in front of the child. This was a more advanced item than the hoop. It shows that the child can follow sound rather than sight.

Each item was a steppingstone to more advanced actions. I began a daily program and I made the trip to St. Paul once a week. It was not easy, but Don and I felt it was important. Lorie needed it, and we didn't want to deny her the good start.

One day, as we were driving to St. Paul, Kathy asked if I would be interested in having Lorie participate in a research project that Jeff was in.

"It is conducted by the University of Minnesota and is a study of Down's Syndrome development. The research staff comes out to the house to do most of the research, but once in awhile they ask you to take your baby to the university for lab tests. They also give I.Q. tests, and I think this is great, since the tests would cost a lot if we had to pay someone to administer one to our babies."

"Do you like being in it?"

"Yes, it's fun, but sometimes I feel a little odd doing the 'Laugh and Smile' items. I like Dante and Linda, the people who are doing most of the work for this study. If I turn your name in, you are under no obligation. If you don't like it, or if you start and change your mind, you can quit any time."

"I guess it wouldn't hurt to look into it. You can give them our name," I answered.

"Good. I think you will like it. First, they will send you a letter explaining more, and then call to see if you are interested. If you are, they will set up an appointment to come out and explain the program to you in more detail."

Life certainly was changing lately. First an Infant Stimulation Program, and now the possibility of participation in a research study.

The letter arrived in the middle of March, asking if Lorie and I would like to be in a study called "Laugh and Smile." "We are studying the affective development in infants with Down's Syndrome."

The letter continued, "The study of affect (smiling, laughter, fear) has been much neglected in child development; yet, we know that emotional-social growth is an equally vital part of development. In fact, it seems most wise to study the total development of the whole child. We hope this is the spirit of our study, as we examine affect expression as a means of determining what the child responds to, experiences and knows."

"What do you think?" I asked Don. "It sounds all right to me. If studying Lorie helps future Down's babies get a good start, it would be worth it."

"Yes, it's okay with me," Don said.

Linda Mans, one of the research staff, called a few days later and set up an appointment for us to meet Dante Cicchetti and learn more about the program.

Dante arrived toward the end of the month with a young man who helped in the program. Dante was a lot younger than I had imagined and looked more like a young student than someone who was conducting most of the research program.

"Mrs. Cobb," he greeted me, "my name is Dante Cicchetti, and I am a graduate student at the university, under the Child Development Program."

After introductions were over and Lorie was admired, Dante continued: "Professor Alan Sroufe and I have been interested in the process of development in

Down's Syndrome infants. The major reason is that while there is a fairly large number of Down's babies born, we know little about their development. What we do know stems mainly from antiquated, stereotyped ideas of what they are like. We want to find out if these are true. Two forty-five-minute visits, arranged at your convenience each month, would be required for each assessment. We will also ask you to come to the university some of the time."

"What will I have to do?"

"It really will not be that hard," he answered. "In the 'Laugh and Smile' part, we have you do some things to see if Lorie will smile, laugh, or whatever.

"As we mentioned in the letter, participation in the research is your choice. If you decide to do it, you can withdraw at any time you wish to.

"At the end of the study," Dante continued, "we will share our findings with you, discuss with you our knowledge concerning play as a means of stimulating development, and provide you with any other information about Lorie that we obtain. Since so little is known about affective development, especially in infants with Down's Syndrome, we do not know how much you might learn about your infant from these exploratory studies. We can make no promises. However, we feel it is vitally important to begin expanding our understanding of these children."

"It sounds all right to us."

"I'm sure you will find it interesting and enjoyable. I will have Linda call you and set up a time for the first appointment. We would like you to come out in the near future for a lab experiment, and we will call you about this."

After Dante and his assistant left, I wondered what it would be like. It certainly would be different than anything I had done before!

My Life Is Changing

Thus says the lord, . . . "Call to Me, and I will answer you, and I will tell you great and mighty things, which you do not know" (Jer. 33:2,3).

The first thing the university asked us to do was participate in an experiment they called the "Loom." We went the following Saturday morning to a stone building marked "The Institute of Child Development."

Dante met us at the doorway, and we followed him to a small room. "You can put Lorie on the table where the baby blanket is," Dante said. "Would you please loosen her clothes so that we can attach a heart monitor to her? We want to check her heartbeat so we can gauge how she is reacting during the testing."

I unsnapped her sleeper and watched Dante as he hooked up the heart monitor. He put a little lubricant on two areas of her chest and placed two small, round, black suction caps over the areas he had lubricated. Around her waist, he attached a small belt that had a transmitter sewn into it. He took the cords that ran from the suction cups and attached them to the transmitter. He taped the loose cords to Lorie's skin and put baby powder over the area.

"I'm finished hooking Lorie up, and you can fasten her outfit," he told me after Linda had verified it was transmitting okay. "As Linda told you on the phone, we are doing this test to see if Lorie will respond defensively to approaching objects. What I want you to do, Mrs. Cobb, is to set Lorie on the stool facing the screen. What will happen," Dante continued, "is that a small diamond-shaped object will get larger and look as if it is going to hit her in the face. We will do this for a few times, and then we will change the position of the diamond and make it look as if it is going to hit her, but it will go off to the side instead."

I watched as Dante, Don, and Kevin left the room. They went into the adjoining room to watch Lorie on the video monitor. Dante switched off the light, and the room darkened. I was apprehensive wondering how Lorie would respond. She was four months old, and one of the youngest babies in this experiment.

I heard a sound that grabbed my attention, and I started watching as a small diamond at the top of the screen started expanding in size. They repeated this several times with an exact time interval between each of the runs. They then switched the course of the diamond, as Dante had told me they would, and the object came down and went off to the side.

My arms were tired, and I hoped the test would be over soon. It seemed that we were there a long time, though I am sure we were there only a few minutes.

The door opened, and Dante turned on the light. "Would you like to come into the other room, and we will run the tape back so that you can see what Lorie did?"

"Yes." Linda had the tape ready and switched it on. We viewed it on a small television monitor, and it was exciting to see little Lorie respond to the object by blinking several times each time it seemed to hit her. When the object moved to the side, Lorie merely tracked it and did not blink. Lorie could obviously discriminate between the two conditions and responded appropriately.

"See—she blinked there." Dante would point at the TV to show us every time she had responded by blinking. "We are finding that Down's Syndrome babies respond similarly to normal babies in this situation."

Dante walked over to the heart monitor and held up the paper with the weird marks on it. "See these marks?" He showed us a specific section of the paper. "Her heartbeat went down, and this shows us she was concentrating then."

Dante had been right: This was interesting and fun to be part of it.

Several days later Dante and Linda came to our house to begin the first "Laugh and Smile" research. We visited for a while before starting the routine that I was to do many more times in the months ahead.

"Now we must ask you to do these things with no response from you, no smiling or whatever. We do not want you to talk to her or do any of the things you usually do when you play with her. Do each item six times with about four-second intervals in between," Dante told me.

I didn't know if I was going to like doing this or not!

"We mark which time she responds to the item; for example, she may smile on trials 2, 5, and 6. We will mark down each item we ask you to do." Dante continued, "Do you have a diaper?"

"Yes." I went into her room to get one.

"Now, Mrs. Cobb," Dante told me, "would you

gently stroke her cheek with it three times? Then, pause four seconds, and repeat it. Do this until you have presented the item six times."

I did as they asked.

I was asked to do various things, like holding a humanlike mask over my face; whispering in her ear, "Hi, baby, how are you?"; blowing gently at her hair for three seconds; and so on, until I had completed fifteen items.

The last item they asked me to do was to crawl across Lorie's field of vision. I was to crawl, stand up, and walk to the place I started from, get back on my knees, and crawl again. Needless to say, I felt foolish doing this and Lorie wasn't even the least bit interested. Actually I felt foolish doing all the items, especially those that called for me to neigh like a horse and say "boo-boo-boo-baa-baa-baa-boo-boo-boo."

Lorie started getting fussy toward the end of the session, and I was glad when they told me this was all they planned to do today. They would complete the last fifteen items the next time they came.

"Some of the items seem so advanced. Why do you have me present them to Lorie now?" I asked Dante and Linda.

"Some of them are advanced, and we do not expect Lorie to respond to them until later. The reason we have you do them now, and in every testing session from now on is that we want to see the exact time she starts to smile, laugh, or even cry with each item."

The list they worked with contained thirty items to be completed in two visits each month. They were broken down into four types: Auditory, Tactile, Social, and Visual. Each time they came they did not follow the list in the same order but would switch around; as their eyes scanned the sheet of paper, they picked out the one they wanted to do next.

My life was changing, and not just in the areas involving Lorie's activities. I didn't really notice it, but one of my girl friends said, "You sure seem different." I wondered, "What is she seeing? Am I really changing?"

Jesus was becoming more and more real to me, and I prayed to Him a lot. My prayers were not said just in a quiet corner or at bedtime, but wherever I was, throwing laundry into the washer, mopping the floor, driving the car. In fact, I had a running conversation with Jesus.

For many years of my life, going to church was a duty, and although I put my time in, I always wished I could really find something there.

I used to go to church each Sunday thinking, "I have to remember God all week, not just at church time." I would kneel before the service started and say prayers to God (which, to me, were sincere).

The service would start, and we would do and say the same things over and over. Thank heaven for the variations—the hymn selections and the different parts of the Gospels that were read to us. The Gospel readings, though they sounded nice, did not make much sense to me. I would find my mind wandering to all the things I wanted to do when we were back home. Deep down in my heart I wished God were more real to us, but He wasn't. Sometimes I wondered if there really was a God, and how I could know for sure. I, at that time, was a professing Christian.

Church suddenly became different—it started with my prayer to Jesus that cold February night. I found myself understanding some of the Gospel lessons and enjoying singing the hymns of praise to Jesus. In fact, I enjoyed going to church now and hated when we had to miss. How different my attitude was from before when it seemed nice when we did not have to go.

And I did not forget God the minute we left the church grounds; He was on my mind constantly. During the week, incidents would cause me to ask questions like: Why does He allow this? What does it mean? Does He say anything about this in the Bible? There was so much I did not know about Jesus, about what the Bible said. As I began questioning more and more, I wanted to start finding the answers.

My reading switched from material about Down's to Christian books—not only were they interesting, but I was learning many things that I had never known before.

One day I went over to a friend's house to visit. I had liked Joy immediately upon meeting her the first day we moved into the neighborhood. She had seemed different to me and more open than most people, and I had sensed she was a good person. I hadn't known why at first, but now I was wondering if it didn't have something to do with Jesus.

I told her about praying to Jesus, and to tell you the truth, I didn't know why I was telling her.

She said, "I wondered if you might have accepted the Lord."

I was happy Joy understood some of what was happening to me and that she was like me. I still didn't understand much of what had happened to me—just that people said I was changing and that Jesus was real to me.

I read my Christian books, and Don saw me reading them. I didn't talk about them, and he never mentioned that my reading material had changed. Maybe he really didn't notice—his life was busy with a job in broadcasting, and the people he worked with were continually calling and asking him about one thing or another. I did not tell him about saying the prayer to Jesus or the fact that Jesus was becoming more and more real to me;

for some reason, I was content with the way things were.

During the first five months of Lorie's life, she was keeping up with her normal counterparts. In May, the chart I was filling out for Dr. Poor read like this: May 2—she rolled from her stomach to her back and picked up a spoon when I placed her hand by it; May 6—she rolled from her stomach to her back, lay there for three or four minutes, and rolled back over the other way.

By the end of May, Lorie had made several accomplishments. When I put fancy shoes on her feet, she really stared at them; she cried when Dad pounded a nail, as it had scared her—she was really noticing the world around her; she transferred an object from one hand to the other and picked up a spoon and grabbed a cup.

We were happy with her progress so far.

Don and I bought her a jump seat like the one at Dr. Poor's, which the physical therapist had put Lorie in as soon as she could hold up her head adequately. She enjoyed it, and by the end of May she was jumping in it very well. She would see her shadow in the doorway and try to jump over it—this kept her occupied for great lengths of time. I loved to watch her!

May's "Laugh and Smile" session found Lorie smiling at some auditory (vocal) items.

On another occasion in May, a member of the research team gave her a developmental test, and I sat on the edge of my chair in a state of nervous apprehension.

When Lorie tried to do an item and couldn't, I would be disappointed.

After the test was completed, the student explained to Don and me that he did not expect Lorie to do all of the items. This was a gauge to see what she could do on different levels, and next time they wanted to see if she could do more. This was used to see how her development was progressing in a number of spheres. Dante wanted to use this as an over-all picture to go with the research items.

At the end of the test the student snapped his fingers to see if Lorie would try to imitate him, and it looked as if she was trying to. This excited Don and me.

I wondered when Lorie would start slowing down. I had noticed the differences in development among the other little ones at Dr. Poor's. Some were advanced, while others were very, very slow. Some in their teen months couldn't even crawl. Of course, I hoped Lorie would be one of the better ones physically.

Don and I also, deep down in our hearts, hoped Lorie would have one of the better I.Q.s, even though special education experts wouldn't really be able to tell until between the ages of two and five years. Some of our expectations, especially in the physical area, were not realistic, and caused us some sorrow later on.

Because Lorie was doing so well, we wanted to keep believing she would continue at this rate.

The month of May brought another first to my life when Eunice, executive director of our county's Association for Retarded Citizens (A.R.C.), called and asked if I would consider doing something.

"Mary Ann, would you like to go with me to the child development class at the Vo-Tech School to speak? I would like you to bring Lorie, show her to the class, and tell them your story. I go there every year and tell the class about the A.R.C. and what we have accomplished.

I didn't know what to think! *Should I do this?* I wondered. *Would I be able to?* My only speaking experience was in school, and it was pure torture!

"The class we will speak to," Eunice continued, "is a

class training for work in Day Care Centers, nurseries, preschools, and for work with handicapped children in special schools. They are covering the section about working with special children, so this is why they would like us to come out now."

Already I was beginning to see the need to educate the public; there were so many misconceptions floating around. If Don and I had been better informed, our finding out about Lorie would not have been quite so hard on us as it was. Because of my strong desire to tell the truth and show others that Lorie and other special children need love, parents to care about them, and all the help possible so that they can live as normally as possible, I consented to do this.

Eunice was pleased that I had agreed to go, and Don was proud of me; however, I was still afraid and nervous.

On the afternoon of our scheduled talk, Eunice picked me up, and we visited on the short trip over to the school.

"Their seeing Lorie will be so much more effective than our talking—in fact, in ways, a lot more effective than words ever could be!" Eunice told me.

The classroom teacher greeted us. "We are so glad you came," she said to me, "and we really appreciate your bringing your baby down here."

The classroom was composed of about twenty young women; the teacher put a chair in the front for Lorie and me to sit in. I was trying not to let my nervousness show. *How will they react? Will they treat us funny? Will they accept us and be glad we came?* All I saw was a sea of faces, and oh, how I hoped they were friendly!

The girls were smiling, and this helped to calm me a bit. They were talking among themselves. "Isn't she cute?" "I wonder how old she is." They were typical young women admiring a small baby.

"Girls," the teacher addressed the class, "this is Eunice . . ."

I didn't hear anything else; my attention got side-tracked by Lorie who was fussing for her bottle. I had brought my electric bottle warmer and plugged it in to heat her bottle.

The bottle quieted Lorie, and Eunice could be heard. She had had a hard time starting out with Lorie's crying.

When Lorie was satisfied, she sat and looked around. She loved all the attention she was getting and decided to make good use of it. Her plan, which worked quite effectively, was to coo, coo, and coo some more.

"I guess," Eunice got out between the coos, "since I am being upstaged, I will let the little lady and her mother have the stage. Mary Ann, would you like to get up and say a few words?"

I stood up. *What in the world was I going to say?* I sent a quick plea to Jesus. Suddenly, a thought flashed across my mind. *Why don't I just visit with them as I would if they were in my living room? After all, this is a very informal deal!*

This is exactly what I did. I told them the sad story from the hospital, how we were adjusting, some things about Dr. Poor's program, and about "Laugh and Smile."

"After the first time the research people came," I told the class, "my husband arrived home in the evening and asked me what I had done and how it went. I told him all the things I had to do to see how Lorie would respond. My husband's comment was,'Who are they testing, you or Lorie?' "

The class laughed at my joke; this was turning out amazingly well! In fact, I was enjoying it, and I had lost my nervousness and found it fun to get some of my points across.

Lorie calmed down, and Eunice resumed her speech in order to finish before the end of class time. The bell rang and the girls came forward, asking if they could hold the baby. Lorie was whisked off and admired by several of them. I received "thank you's" for coming by almost the whole class—this made it worthwhile giving up one of my afternoons.

The teacher visited with us and told us a couple of her students were receiving some of their training in the Day Activity Center and were learning a lot by working with the mentally retarded youngsters. I went home happy I had done this.

A View
of the Future

And you shall know the truth, and the truth shall make you free (John 8:32).

Mary called me one evening and asked if we would like to come out Sunday and meet Nancy, a nineteen-year-old Down's Syndrome girl. Don and I accepted the invitation and looked forward to going.

The more we could see of Down's children older than Lorie, the more we would know what Lorie's future would be like.

Nancy came into Pat and Mary's life when they decided to take a foster child into their home. She arrived to join the family in September of 1969 when she was fourteen.

"We looked for someone near Sandy's age," Mary told me. "We applied for a Down's child, since we knew something about this handicap. We got Nancy when her foster mother wanted to find a different home for her. The lady was an older lady and felt that Nancy was too much responsibility for her."

"Nancy," Mary continued, "worked out very well for us, because she was independent and self-sufficient. She was well-mannered and well-behaved. In fact, we really had only one troublesome problem with her, and that was that she went into the kitchen and snitched food!"

"When you think of all the problems she could have caused, she really wasn't bad, was she?" I questioned.

"No, not at all," Mary answered me. "Nancy has always been a proud girl and takes pride in her appearance. She was a lot of help around the house; she loves to do domestic things."

"Did she go to school near you?" I asked.

"Yes, she was bused to the public school and was in a trainable, special education class."

"When did she leave you?"

"She left in November of 1974 to live in the Community Living Group Home."

"Were you sad to see her go?" (If I were a foster mother, I'm sure I would become so attached, it would be hard to see the child leave.)

"No. I said I would never be sad to see her go to a better place. If she had gone to a worse place or into an institution, I would have cried. I was happy to see her go to the group home, as it is perfect for her and good for her to be with her peers. There are a lot of fun things to do when they are not working."

"Was Nancy ever in an institution?"

"Yes, for five years. After she came to live with us we had a hard time working out some of her institution traits. She hung her head and would never look us in the eyes. People who come out of institutions often have many negative body language signs, as Nancy did."

"Lorie and Sandy are lucky they are growing up in their homes," I commented.

"Yes, and they will probably look a lot better because they have a chance to use all their muscles. Some of the children in institutions do not use all their muscles, especially the facial muscles. If they try to talk, often it's in vain since no one listens to them."

Our meeting Nancy turned out to be a positive encounter for us. "What do you think about Nancy?" I asked my husband on the drive home.

"She is such a nice girl," he said, "I hope we can rear Lorie to turn out as well as Nancy."

"I hope we can, too," I answered. I thought about our visit as Don drove us home that cool, spring evening.

Nancy turned out to be a lot different than I had expected! She was an attractive young woman with short, blonde hair. She was dressed neatly in slacks and a top, and did not look much different from a normal nineteen-year-old, although you could tell she was Down's.

Nancy had a pleasant smile, and she came over and asked to hold Lorie; Nancy loved babies.

Though her development wasn't at the level of a normal nineteen-year-old, she was functioning well, and Don and I were pleased to see what a useful person she was. We were able to see that Lorie could have a future, too, and that she would be able to do things. This reassured us. One of our biggest fears was that Lorie would be so slow in functioning that she would require constant care the rest of our lives.

"Both participating in the programs for Down's Syndrome children and seeing how well Nancy was doing helped us to see that Lorie could have a useful life in the world. We had a positive goal to work for—Lorie could contribute to the world if we gave her the chance!

Not long after our visit with Nancy, the physical therapist working with Dr. Poor came out to do an evaluation on Lorie; the test measured Lorie at twenty weeks old. This meant she was not behind in her physical development at this stage of her life.

The physical therapist began working with Lorie on how to balance herself. She wanted Lorie to use arm extension to catch herself when she leaned to one side and to push herself back up. The therapist would push Lorie quickly to one side, trying to build up Lorie's reaction to use her arm to stop the fall.

The sheet Lorie was working on now dealt with what she would do with a mirror (she was a ham!); whether or not she would pick a cube off the table; how she would do if I handed her three cubes.

The three blocks confused her. She always wanted the third cube even though she had two cubes in her hands, and this frustrated her. Dr. Poor wanted to know if Lorie would approach the third cube to try to take hold of it, even if she couldn't actually get the cube.

Many times during the sessions, Dr. Poor would give the group helpful information. Once she told us, "Your children's toys should have a purpose. These toys should do something for the child and not just be something to play with!"

I could see her point: A toy with a purpose helps in the teaching and development of our children.

July came, bringing hot weather. Lorie continued doing well in her development. She completed the seven-month chart the first part of the month—she was keeping up with her age development so far.

One thing Dr. Poor had asked me to do with Lorie at home was to giver her dry Cheerios cereal. She wanted Lorie to pick them up with the first finger and thumb to develop her pincher grip. This hard for Lorie, and we were finding out that fine motor development was something she was having trouble with. I kept putting the Cheerios out for her, even though most of the time she picked them up wrong. By the end of the month, she had managed to use her thumb and finger a couple of times.

One day Lorie sat up at Dr. Poor's for over a half hour; everyone made a fuss over this! Lorie enjoyed the attention. One of the mothers, whose child sat up much later, commented that it was nice Lorie was sitting up already.

Yes, I thought to myself, *how lucky we are that she is doing okay physically*.

How naïve I had been that day. It never entered my mind that she would slow down physically and others would pass her by!

In September the physical therapist started working with Lorie on crawling and getting up and down from a sitting position by herself. To teach crawling, the therapist put Lorie on a little board with wheels; it looked like a skate board. She would lay Lorie on her stomach and put her arms and legs over the sides. The physical therapist wanted Lorie to use her arms and legs to move it. Lorie did not like this at all!

Kathy and I decided to organize a mothers' group in our county. We did so with the help of the A.R.C. Our first meeting was held in September, and we had a very good turn out. I found out how important it is to have fellowship with other Down's mothers and to be able to share freely concerning our common experience.

I had never thought about how fortunate we had been to get Lorie into programs right away until I met Gail. I came into contact with her through my doctor and had found out that she was the mother of a sixteen-month-old Down's girl. Her daughter Stacie was doing well in her development, considering she had not been in early programs.

Gail had never heard about early intervention programs and was surprised that Lorie had been receiving help since she was a small baby. I put Gail in contact with Dante, and he was able to help her find a program for Stacie.

Many changes were taking place in our household since Lorie's birth. But in the fall, another big change occurred, unrelated to Lorie's problems, that helped bring Don and I closer to the Lord.

Don was unhappy with his job, and he was growing more unhappy each day. Everything about our recent move to the Twin Cities had worked out, except our reason for moving—Don's job.

With money tight, there was always the fear the cable television company Don worked for would stop broadcasting altogether. Don lived with the uncertainty that his job might not be there the next day. Besides that, the job was very demanding time-wise. Not only did he have to spend long hours there , but when he was home the telephone rang constantly with pleas for help: "Don, how do you fix this? The sound went off!" We were never free of the demands of the job.

I remember one incident in particular that helped trigger Don's decision to look for other employment. A group of parents with Down's children formed a parents' group, which we started attending. Don and I were there one evening for a couple of hours (it took us an hour to drive there), when someone from Don's office called. Because of some serious technical problems, we had to leave in the middle of the meeting, and both Don and I were unhappy about this.

One evening soon after that, I mentioned the possibility of his looking for another job.

"I guess you're right," Don agreed. "I think I'll start looking for one right away."

His job hunting did not prove fruitful as soon as we would have liked. Several days after he had started looking, just after we had retired for the evening, Don expressed his disappointment in not finding another job yet.

"Why don't you pray to Jesus and ask Him to help you find a job?" I surprised myself by saying this to him!

I wondered if he was stunned. He answered, "I guess so."

"Would you like to pray to Him aloud?" I asked.

"No, I really don't know how to pray aloud. I don't know what to say."

"I can help you this time if you want me to."

"Yes, please."

"Dear Jesus, Don is very unhappy with his job. Would You please help him find a better one?" The room was silent, and I wondered what Don would do.

Then slowly and carefully Don started to pray —it was a beautiful prayer, as he reached out in faith to Jesus.

We were on our way home from church the next Sunday when Don felt impressed to get a Sunday newspaper. He turned the car around and headed for a store where they had a newspaper stand.

At home, he sat in his white recliner, and started looking through the want ads for a job. His eyes came across an ad for a TV service manager. He quickly passed it by and started looking in the ads in the broadcasting area. His eyes seemed to be pulled back to that ad. He again went back to the broadcasting listings. Again, his eyes turned to this small ad. He was puzzled. Then he thought, *Maybe Someone is trying to tell me this is the job He wants me to have!*

Don applied for the job on Monday. The man hiring was very pleased with Don's qualifications, which met every one they wanted, including experience with video tape. "I can't make the final hiring until the man from the main office comes. We will call you in for another interview when he is here," he said.

Don was called at the end of the week.

"I don't have time to change. Can I come in my work clothes?" Don wore a uniform.

"Yes, come as soon as possible. The man from the main office will be here only a few hours."

Don asked to leave his job early and drove over for the second interview. He came home to tell me the news.

"Mary Ann, the job is mine. Would you believe I beat ten guys out of that job!"

We were happy; the job sounded good, and the hours were better, and so was the pay. The only disadvantage was that he would have to travel from time to time. Don started his new job in December and loved it.

He could never say exactly what day he started trusting the Lord, but when he saw that the Lord answered prayers and could provide a good job, he believed.

One Christian friend gave me some cassette tapes her minister had recorded. Listening to good Bible teaching showed me that Don and I needed to be in a Bible study and learn more about what the Bible says.

One night, I asked Don at supper if we could go to the Friday night Bible study held in my friend's home.

"Okay, it sounds fine with me."

Joy, my Christian neighbor, took our children, and we drove there on a cold December evening.

The minister, a man in his early thirties, taught on the Gospel of John that evening. Don and I were amazed to see how much could be learned from the Bible. The minister kept having us search through the Bible for verses that tied in with what he was teaching.

We, with our very, very little Bible teaching, had a hard time finding the places. There was no doubt we had a lot to learn!

Don was pleased with being taught about the Bible and said it reminded him of Bible teaching he had had at the beginning of his Sunday school life.

"Do you want to keep going?" I asked him.

"What a question!" he answered emphatically. "Yes, I want to."

How our lives were changing! Jesus was putting us on a different path to live our lives; He was starting to teach us. Don and I both knew we had to go forward, and learning His way would help us do this.

An Unrealistic Dream

In everything give thanks; for this is God's will for you in
Christ Jesus (I Thess. 5:18).

I had a big dream for Lorie. It really was an unrealistic dream, but nevertheless I had it. I wanted Lorie to
develop as well as the little girl in the films we had
watched.

This dream started shortly after Lorie was born when
the health nurse sent Don and me to see some films
about an infant stimulation program in a nearby
county. At this time, Lorie was not yet in Dr. Poor's
program.

"I think," the health nurse had told me during one of
her visits, "it will be helpful for you two to see what a
stimulation program is like and what it is able to accomplish."

The film was shown in the house of one of the
couples whose child was in the program. A cute little
dark-haired girl about eighteen months old greeted us
at the door with her mother. We learned she had been
born with chromosome errors in the number thirteen
match-up.

Lorie

The lady who headed the stimulation program was the one showing the films. A young woman in her early thirties, she became interested in this work because she had two mentally retarded sons.

She visited freely with the parents with whose children she worked. "Your son is doing so much better. He has improved since I saw him last week," she told the parents of a brain-damaged boy.

"Do you really think so?" the mother exclaimed.

"Yes, you will notice the improvement on the films from the first time we worked with him until now."

The first film she showed us was of her working with this boy. Don and I were utterly amazed at how much was involved in working with him. The film showed two years of working with him, with shots taken at intervals; it wasn't until the end of the film that they were working with him on how to sit up.

The therapist was talking as the film was running, and we learned that the boy was not only brain damaged but also paralyzed on one side and blind!

The next film was of her working with a brain-damaged girl who was also partially paralyzed and blind. The little boy was doing better than she was.

The film showing the work with the little Trisomy 13 girl was interesting. We learned that this is a very rare handicap. A lot of chromosome errors in the teen numbers result in death either before or right after birth.

"We did not know what kind of a program to set up for her, because we do not really know what her handicap involves. We finally decided to put her through the Down's Syndrome program," the therapist said.

To Don and I, the little girl appeared to be doing well; she was walking before the age of two.

The film that interested us the most was the one where the therapist worked with a little Down's Syndrome girl. It showed her working with the girl from the time she was a tiny baby up to almost the age of two.

"Doesn't Lorie look like her?" I whispered to Don. She looked the same age as Lorie was at that time.

"Yes," Don whispered back. "It's as if we are looking at our baby and not someone else's."

"This little girl," the therapist told the small group, "is developing the same as her normal counterpart and has not slowed down yet. We are excited and are trying to push her ahead as much as possible before she starts to slow down."

We were excited to see a Down's child that was doing well—in fact, she didn't seem different from any other child her age.

Don and I were interested in what differences there were between Lorie and the little girl who had been born Trisomy 13. Her mother told us that her child had a hearing problem (she wore a hearing aid), no finger and toe prints, and a malformed nose. Her chromosome error is rare, and doctors do not know all that could be involved physically. Her parents were taking her life a day at a time.

The evening had been an interesting one, and we were able to see that there were parents who were facing greater difficulties than we were.

"The little girl born Trisomy 13 was sure a little darling, wasn't she?" I said to Don on the way home.

"Yes, I got a kick out of how she loved showing off for everyone there."

As I thought back over the exceptional development of the little Down's girl in the film, I began to dream of Lorie's developing the same way. Then when Lorie started out doing well, I psyched myself into believing she was going to do just as well as the little girl in the film had.

When Lorie first enrolled in Dr. Poor's programs, the

physical therapist gave each of us mothers a chart on motor development, which Dr. Poor later added to her book.[3] I always looked at the chart to see how Lorie was coming on development, and looked to see if her development was normal. The chart said the normal age for sitting alone is seven months. Lorie did this on schedule. She was keeping up with her normal peers.

Now that she could sit up, I was anxious for her to be able to get up and back down by herself. I was sure it would not be long before she could do this. Though I knew Down's babies were slower, I believed she was going to keep doing as well as she had in the past.

The physical therapist started working on this right after Lorie mastered sitting up. She would hold tightly to the upper part of Lorie's leg and teach her how to use her arms to push herself up from the side.

At home, I worked and worked with Lorie on this stimulation. I wanted her to do it as soon as possible. My working with her did not seem to be doing much good—she was not catching on as I thought she should. Some days tears ran down my face after an unproductive work session.

As the days continued with no real response, a nagging thought kept running across my mind: *Lorie is getting behind in her physical development—she is not doing well.*

One day, after the physical therapist had completed working with Lorie, I mentioned how Lorie did not seem to be picking this up. "She is starting to do it a little if I get her started," I said.

"She probably is not ready yet, and you are trying to push her too fast. Keep working with her, but don't drive yourself wild doing it. She will do it when *she* is ready."

The therapist was right! I had been pushing Lorie and

expecting something from her that she could not yet do. I had to start facing the fact that she probably wasn't going to be exceptional like that Down's girl who developed almost normally in both physical and mental development.

My bubble was bursting; Lorie *was* falling behind in her physical development. How hard it was to admit that I had undue expectations for her! Time had a way of showing me I had to let go of this unrealistic dream. I could see now that Lorie *was* much slower than normal babies her age.

Normal babies who were Lorie's age could do things that she was unable to do, and they did them easily. Lorie's accomplishments came after lots and lots of hard work. Sometimes this fact would make me upset or depressed, and my mind would scream, *It's not fair! That baby does things on his own while everything is so hard for Lorie!*

Don and I both realized how much we had taken for granted with Kevin. We were happy and proud when he did new things, but we never realized how much of a miracle it really was!

I had jealous feelings toward parents with normal babies who were near Lorie's age. I tried to shove these feelings aside rather than admit them. Coming to terms with Down's means accepting all that it involves. Lorie was Down's, and she was going to lag behind the normal child; she wasn't going to be the exceptional Down's I had wanted her to be.

It is said that growing hurts, and I believe it. It hurts to face the facts, pick up the pieces, and go on from there.

Rumors circulated in the fall that money might not be allotted to continue Dr. Poor's program. A lot of us hoped it would continue, since it would be awhile before our children could enter the Day Activity Centers.

Dr. Poor had started her program four years earlier, and during the time she worked with the children, she gathered information to write a book about her work. The book was written and at the publisher; it was doubtful the research money would be allotted any longer. Dr. Poor had accomplished her purpose for starting the program.

In December the verdict came; this program would be terminated at the end of the month.

Dr. Poor gave a Christmas party; it was also a going-away party. I took both Kevin and Lorie to it.

The big attraction at the party was Dr. Poor's book, which had just arrived from the publisher. I found Lorie's picture right away; it had been taken when she had first entered the program. In the picture, the physical therapist was working with Lorie to teach her to hold her head up. In the parents' section, I found the small piece I had written, which told how I had been informed of Lorie's handicap. One section in the book was devoted to Dante's "Laugh and Smile" research program.

It was exciting to know that we were part of a book to help new parents get the right information. This book also showed what an infant stimulation program was like and that early intervention was indeed helping.

I bought a copy for us and a few for our relatives. The other mothers were buying several copies, too, and the supply quickly dwindled.

Dr. Poor had worked with thirty-three children, and the surprising thing was that most of us mothers were young. A chart in the book broke down the age groupings of us mothers whose children had been involved in the program. The chart was based on our age when our child was born.[4]

17-24 years of age	20.60%
25-29 years of age	34.40%
30-34 years of age	31.03%
35-39 years of age	6.90%
40-44 years of age	6.90%
45 plus	0%

Many of us were under thirty when we had our Down's baby. I was twenty-eight when I had Lorie. One of the mothers in the group was nineteen and a first-time mother when her Down's son was born.

It's true that the older you get, the higher your chances are of having a Down's,[5] but more and more younger mothers are having them. It used to be thought this was just something that happened to older mothers.

At the party, I met some of the mothers who went to sessions on different days than the one I took Lorie to. It was nice to meet them, see their little ones, and show each other our child's picture in Dr. Poor's book.

The Christmas season was fast approaching, and the closer the holiday came, the more I realized I was not looking forward to it. I went through the routine of getting ready, but only half-heartedly.

Don and I were going to be away from our relatives this Christmas, the first time in a few years, and we did not have much planned.

I did invite some neighbors (Roger, Linda, Missy, and Matthew) over to celebrate Lorie's first birthday. Lorie didn't know what to think about packages for her, angel food cake, and people singing "Happy Birthday" to her! Afterward, she loved playing with the gifts, boxes, and wrapping paper.

At six o'clock, Christmas Eve, it became evident why I had not looked forward to Christmas: I was remembering last year's events. In each time period, I was reliving the year before! At eight o'clock, I remembered opening the gifts; at 10:15, they were putting me in my room, and on and on.

This is awful! I thought, but try as I might, I was not able to get my mind off this subject! Being alone for Christmas did not turn out to be such a good thing. There was nothing to detract my attention. I kept dwelling on last year.

This was dragging Don down, too, though he didn't seem to be showing it as much as I was.

"Don," I told him Christmas Day, "we should have gone away for the holiday. If we would have had other things on our minds, we would not have had so much time to wallow in self-pity!"

Don agreed that next year we should be with our relatives and friends.

I called my friend Mary, Sandy's mother, right after the holiday season to tell her about how depressed we had been and to ask if she had this problem around Sandy's birthday.

"Yes, it bothered us for about the first five years, but now we don't give much thought to it. It will get better each year."

I was thankful to have Mary for a friend! She answered all my questions, encouraged me when I was down, and shared my excitement with Lorie's new accomplishments. Mary's reassurance helped me to face the situation.

With the holiday season out of the way, the Lord started teaching Don and me His ways. Up to now, our walk with the Lord had been nurtured through our prayers and His gentle guiding, and we followed Him in childlike faith. When Don and I entered the Friday-night fellowship and started being taught what God's Word said, we had a strong desire to read. I spent every extra minute I could find with a book in front of me. I wanted to learn as much as I could about the Lord.

I borrowed some of our minister's cassette tapes to listen to his Bible teachings. I listened as I mopped floors, washed dishes, and did other household chores.

How excited I was to learn what had happened when I prayed my prayer to Jesus several months before. I learned salvation is from the Lord!

How often in earlier years, before I had accepted Christ, had I wondered if I was going to heaven. What if I didn't? I shuddered to think of it. I knew I was a sinner and I had things in my past that I was ashamed of. "But," I always rationalized, "I'm not as bad as so-and-so, and I haven't done some of the awful sins some people do! I am trying to do better. Surely the Lord will not put me in hell for trying to do my best. I'm really not that bad, am I?"

Still, I did not have any assurance that I would go to heaven.

Much of my religious life had been centered on trying to keep the law. I wanted to obey the rules and be a perfect person, but somehow I never managed. I couldn't make the grade. But I wouldn't admit I was a bad person.

I wanted to be Christian, but somehow my Christian life didn't go very well. The more hopeless it became to live up to what I thought I should be, the more discouraged I was. My mind would tell me, *I'm not going to heaven. I just know it. I can't measure up.* I was a mixed-up mess.

Maybe this is one of the reasons why Don and I didn't go to church when we were first married. After I became pregnant with Kevin, we both felt we needed to go to church so that Kevin could have religious training.

We started attending a church, but God wasn't real to either of us. We just made the effort to get there and endure the service. My going to church was a way of reassuring myself that I was a Christian. If there was a God, I was showing Him I was in church to worship Him. It was like a safeguard to protect me if there really was a God. How wrong I was; this changed the day I asked Jesus into my heart.

I learned that going to church doesn't save you, and that there was no possible way for my salvation to have come through keeping rules. God's standard to be saved by the law is shown in Matthew 5:48: "Therefore you are to be perfect, as your heavenly Father is perfect." This I could not have done. I later learned that if you commit even one sin, God considers you guilty of the whole law.

In Romans 3:10,23, I learned that "there is none righteous, not even one; . . . for all have sinned and fall short of the glory of God." God was telling me that there isn't a single man who is able to keep the law and never sin.

Romans 6:23 showed me what God's penalty for sin is: "For the wages of sin is death, but the free gift of God is eternal life in Christ Jesus our Lord."

Salvation does not come through works (law), but through believing in Jesus and accepting His free gift of salvation.

Ephesians 2:8,9 reads, "For by grace you have been saved through faith; and that not of yourselves, it is the gift of God; not as a result of works, that no one should boast."

The Scriptures taught me He saves when you believe in Him.

Romans 10:9 reads, "If you confess with your mouth Jesus as Lord, and believe in your heart that God raised Him from the dead, you shall be saved."

First Peter 1:23 says, "For you have been born again [born from above] not of seed which is perishable but imperishable, *that is*, through the living and abiding word of God." Born again, I learned from the taped sermons and Bible teaching, means regenerated by the Holy Spirit operating through the Word of God.

"The Jews," the minister explained on the tape, "used to think they were saved because they were born in Abraham's blood line, but God says no. We are not saved by this way or by any of the works men do trying to save themselves. We are born by God." What freedom in knowing I did not have to make the grade! Salvation comes from God!

I had never really thought about the Cross and how God loved us enough to work out a plan for saving fallen humanity. The plan was His Son Jesus, who became sin in our behalf. Jesus was the perfect sacrifice for our sins.

The Cross is the answer! Our salvation doesn't come through our own merit, but by Jesus Christ. How lucky we are that God cared enough about us to send His Son to die on the cross in our place. Through what Jesus did, we can come to God.

Don and I were starting to understand the freedom of belonging to the Lord and of being forgiven of all our sins. Christ died on the cross for *all* our sins, past, present, and future. Our old sin nature was taken to the cross with Jesus, and now we are free to walk and grow in Him. Romans 8:1 tells us how free we are: "There is therefore now no condemnation for those who are in Christ Jesus."

Since we received Him by grace through faith, we are to walk in grace (seeking God's will in everything and trusting in Him) by faith. Without the terrible fear of what the Lord would do, and with the freedom of knowing we were forgiven and there was no condemnation, Don and I set out on the road ahead that He was leading us on.

Would He teach us some of the reasons why He gave Lorie to us? We hoped so.

One Beautiful Reason

. . . always being ready to make a defense to every one who asks you to give an account for the hope that is in you, yet with gentleness and reverence (1 Pet. 3:15).

Life seemed different now that Kathy and I were no longer making the weekly trip to Dr. Poor's. It seemed as if there were a void in my life! I missed the instruction sheets that mapped out a work program for Lorie and the helpful suggestions from the physical therapist.

One morning I called our county health nurse. "Have you organized a group program yet?" A year had passed since we last talked.

The answer was discouraging. "No, but we can come out to your house if you want us to."

"Could you bring the physical therapist, too?" I inquired.

"Yes, when would it be convenient?"

We set up a time, and when they came to our home later that same day, they showed me some new things to include in my work program for Lorie.

I no longer *pushed* Lorie beyond her obvious

capabilities. My working with her was to *encourage* her to do things but *not to force* her. She was going to learn in her own time.

Dante, the young man who headed the research program Lorie was in, told me one day, "There are some things you can work on and some things that you have to wait for until the child can work on it."

Dante Cicchetti and Alan Sroufe have an article that appears in Dr. Poor's book, and they elaborate on this concept:

> Sensitivity, responsivity, and cooperativeness are requirements for all caregivers interacting with infants. Caregivers need to be alert to the infant's cues; for example, they must note whether the baby's attention is waning or if it needs to break contact temporarily. They must respond to the infant's signals of pleasure or distress and changes in mood. Often, they must create the climate in which mutually rewarding interaction can occur, *making sure that the intervention is timely and not abrupt.*
>
> Caregivers of Down's Syndrome infants are called upon to extend themselves much more than the typical caregiver. . . . Helping these infants sustain attention and build excitement is especially challenging. Young Down's Syndrome infants are less responsive by temperament, and their cues or signals are minimally visible. They are difficult to "read" and relatively unexpressive; for example, because of a relative lack of muscle tone, their facial expressions are often subtle and not well differentiated. They are not quick to respond to inputs from their caregivers. All of these factors place a burden on the caregiver to be physically cuddly, to generate and maintain lively interchanges, and to stay actively involved with the infant in the absence of typical feedback and input from the baby.[6]

If I had known some of this information. I wouldn't have beat my head against the wall trying to get Lorie to do something she wasn't able to do. I would have looked for cues in her response and gone from there. I could have accepted that she wasn't ready to sit up by herself!

Lorie was a passive baby, and the fact she did not protest to her mother's obsession to get her to sit up by herself *did not help!* Just as indicated above, she did not give me many cues. My attempts were futile. (Why is it that hindsight is always better than foresight?)

How carefree our work times had become now that I was no longer struggling with it. If she seemed tired or uninterested, I was willing to quit and leave my working with her until she was more receptive.

On Friday nights Don and I continued to go to the Bible study group we had joined. We were hungry to learn what the Bible said, and we enjoyed the Christian fellowship.

One evening the minister's teaching entered the subject of suffering. "The believer's suffering is to show that he is learning lessons," he said.

How true. We were learning from our suffering. I listened as he explained that "the unbeliever's suffering is to bring him to the Lord."

Don was looking up the Scripture reference that the minister had given, but my mind was wandering. Something had clicked for me in that last statement. *Is this why He gave us Lorie? Was it to reach us?* My mind began a mad race backward—a flood of scenes filled my mind. In fact, I was feeling some of the sad emotions that had occurred then. *How I had suffered when I had been told about Lorie! What a shock the news had brought!*

Feelings of helplessness, of being almost devastated, had engulfed me at that time. It had caused me to begin my search that led to accepting Jesus.

Oh, we had had other traumas and misfortunes in

our lives, but this was the first one we hadn't been able to solve on our own. Though Don had adjusted faster than I had, it still affected both of our lives.

It had indeed taken a radical incident to reach us! If Lorie hadn't come to us, would we still have accepted Jesus, or would we still be heading on our merry way in a life without Jesus? Thank heaven He threw the very things in front of me that I couldn't handle. It was this factor that had gotten me to call on Jesus that cold February night.

I wondered how many other times Jesus had tried to reach us through incidents, but we had rejected Him. There was no doubt He had gotten my attention with Lorie's arrival!

Excitement filled me as I realized just one small reason why He had permitted us to have Lorie. He did not give us Lorie out of anger. He loved and cared for us so much that He had found a way to reach us!

The month of February found Don on a plane heading for Chicago concerning his job, and the kids and me in a car heading for my sister's home in Iowa. In the last months I had started talking more freely about Jesus, and on this visit I talked with my sister and her husband about Him.

My sister listened; she had learned some of the same things in a previous Bible study, though she had not made a commitment to Jesus. I was able to talk with my brother-in-law when I watched a late TV movie with him. The movie was about a man conducting a séance. He was trying to contact someone who had lived in the 1800s. This was a movie that I would not have watched had I been home!

It wasn't too long after the program began when I exclaimed, "That man is mixed up in the occult!" This grabbed Bruce's attention. "I read somewhere that people conducting séances aren't talking to the dead, but to demons disguised as the departed. Being mixed up in the occult is bad, and in Hal Lindsey's book *Satan Is Alive and Well on Planet Earth* he talks about that from a Christian point of view."

How ironic that the things I shared with my brother-in-law were things I had learned from some of my own experiences. I now wanted to share God's answer for today's world, salvation through His Son Jesus Christ.

After the visit at my sister's, the children and I went to Rochester to visit relatives and friends. During this visit I was more free to talk about Lorie's handicap. I told most of the people I had worked with in Rochester about Lorie. This was a big step, as I expected negative reactions. But to my amazement, I didn't receive any. Since people did not reject the news about Lorie, I was encouraged to tell more and more people.

Our friends who had known about Lorie from the beginning were feeling free to ask questions. They would ask, "Does it bother you to answer these questions?" "Do you mind?" Don and I (Don had joined me in Rochester) would reassure them that it did not bother us, and we liked to answer questions as openly and truthfully as we could. This, we felt, was an excellent way to educate the public and correct misconceptions.

We were positive in our answers concerning Lorie and what her handicap involved. I think this had a lot to do with people accepting her. Even people we met for the first time responded positively.

For quite awhile I had wondered why people hadn't responded negatively when we told them Lorie had been born with Down's Syndrome. I had, in a way, prepared myself for negative reactions and was stunned when I did not receive them—not even once!

One day the reason for this dawned on me: We

painted a positive outlook. We often told people of good programs being offered and about these children becoming useful citizens in our world. Because of this, people picked up our positive attitudes!

I am in no way saying we are always 100 percent positive—this just isn't true! We are human; we have our down days, and I often fight to overcome depression. Some days things just seem harder than other days. But most of the time we have a positive outlook concerning our daughter.

What a big growth step Jesus had taken me on when He helped me realize that our attitudes make a difference in how people respond to us—and to Lorie!

Another thing that I was beginning to realize is that Jesus is using our little daughter to help change Don and me from rough rocks into precious stones! We are learning from her, and I hope we can teach her to be a happy, responsible person who knows how much Jesus loves her.

When we first were told about Lorie, we thought it was the worst thing that had ever happened to us. Now Jesus was showing us that it wasn't. He was turning this situation around and using it for our good. Jesus causes all things to work together for good and for His glory (see Rom. 8:28).

When we returned to Minneapolis I went to the regular meeting of Down's mothers. How much I enjoyed this get-together and seeing the new accomplishments of the little ones. How proud we all were when our children showed off their newly mastered feats!

A couple of the children were getting near the age to enter the Day Activity Center; they looked so small to board a school bus and be whisked off to school. In another year, Lorie would be going—how fast time was flying!

The topic of conversation changed to a serious note

when one of the mothers said, "You know, having a handicapped child really humbles you!"

After thinking about what this mother had said, I started writing about what Lorie was teaching me.

How proud parents can be when their child arrives "normal"—they want to show their baby off to everyone! They are sure this is the world's cutest and smartest baby. They are sure he is going to be something extra special in the world, a famous doctor, or whatever they dream about. When their child does some new feat, the parents know this is showing how smart and talented their child is.

As time goes on, they find out their child may not be the cutest or the smartest, but he or she is "normal" and does have a good chance in this world. They have an idea of what the future holds for the child—college or trade school, marriage, and maybe a job the child will really like.

But when the baby arrives who isn't perfect by the world's standard, how it changes its parents' lives! They can't brag that their baby is the cutest or the smartest—their smooth world has hit a ruffle! They suddenly have to deal with all that is involved in coping with and rearing a special baby. Not only does it change what they say to the world, but it forces them to think about what is important.

As Chris Byroads, who was to soon enter Lorie's life as her music therapist, so adequately states, "Things you once thought were so important will not matter anymore! Your whole world has changed!"

We aren't telling the world that Lorie is cute (she has the Down's features) or smart (she's retarded). We think she's cute, but we are her parents. We can't brag that she did things sooner than someone else—in fact, she doesn't always do things as well as some of the other Down's children!

We do have normal parental pride. We are happy when Kevin brings home a star paper from school and when Lorie finally does what we have been working with her on. We usually tell our friends when Lorie has learned something new. The day she learned how to get up into a sitting position by herself, I called several people. Now, I wasn't gloating. I was just glad she had finally learned it. For her, everything comes after lots of work, and we are proud when she learns something new—not because she is better than anyone else's child now—but because it is truly an accomplished feat.

Jesus is teaching us lessons on humility through our tiny daughter. How exciting it is to learn that He uses many everyday incidents to teach us what He desires us to learn!

Chris, a vivacious, enthusiastic and optimistic young woman, became Lorie's music therapist.

At the mothers' group we had been told that Chris was opening a music therapy program for little ones. The only requirement was that they be able to sit up.

That evening, when Don arrived home, I presented the idea of Lorie being in it. "It would be two half-hour sessions a week, and the cost is only five dollars a week."

"That's reasonable. Where will the sessions be held?"

"In one of the mother's homes. What do you think?"

"It sounds okay to me," Don told me. "I liked what we saw of her program. Why don't you call her and say that we are interested?"

I was *so* excited—Lorie was going to be in an organized program again. I knew this one was going to be fun from the things Don and I had learned when Chris gave a talk for the A.R.C.

We had gone one evening in the fall. Our first view of Chris was from the back of a large room with about seventy other people. She was a petite young woman with a bubbly personality that came through as she began the first few minutes of her talk.

"My name is Chris Byroads, and I am a music therapist. I'm sure many of you have not heard of music therapy, so let me give you a little introduction to what it is. Music therapy is a relatively new field and became widely used after World War II because of its effectiveness with hospitalized veterans. Music therapy was first offered as a degree at the University of Michigan in 1950. When the National Association of Music Therapy was created under the direction of Dr. E. Thayer Gaston in Lawrence, Kansas, music therapy became closely associated with the University of Kansas located in Lawrence. During the past ten years, as people became more aware of its value, music therapy has been given degree status in a number of universities. Because music therapy is flexible and easily individualized, it is effective with all handicaps, whether emotional, physical, or intellectual, and can be used with people of all ages."

Chris was talking not only to a group of parents of retarded children but also to people who work with the retarded and to a few young retarded people. (It was nice to know that the young retarded people were included in the membership meetings.)

"The music therapist," Chris continued, "has an extensive background in the areas of psychology, special education, and physical handicaps. They are taught to adapt music to individual problems and to help people work through their problems or handicaps in a nonthreatening environment.

"Our music therapy program is for children in special education or children who have learning or emotional problems that require special attention. It is designed to add another dimension to the current treatment of your child's learning or behavioral problem. It provides an enjoyable success experience for children while strengthening and developing their learning skills.

"If you decide to put your child in the program, much of the success of the program will depend on your interest and participation. Often you will be asked to join us and assist in the sessions. Your praise and opinion of your child's work is always invaluable."

Chris explained some of the things she did in working with the children; her students varied in age from three years to teen-age. She also told about the various instruments she used in working with her charges: autoharp, songbells, melodica, organ, drum, and guitar. I marveled that little handicapped children could learn to play these things.

We were delighted when she played a cassette tape of two little boys she was working with to show how they were learning to get along. It was sweet to hear them talking to each other.

"Some of the other goals we work on are conversation, friendships, socializing, and learning. The child is given the opportunity to enjoy learning, and the child controls the pace. No child is spoonfed information. The child is always aware when he understands a new concept, and he is proud of his new ability."

The program certainly sounded good—if Lorie was old enough, we would consider putting her in. At this time, Chris had not said that she worked with babies.

"Developing a good self-image, self-esteem, and self-confidence *is a very, very important goal,* Chris continued. "I work with the children until (1) each activity is successful, (2) each child is successful, (3) each child feels good about his successes, and (4) each child feels good about himself."

I was to learn how important self-esteem is when I read Dr. James Dobson's book, *Hide and Seek*. Low self-esteem, according to Dobson, is a big problem in our country, and he gives some ideas for parents to help a child gain self-esteem. Low self-esteem is a problem for me, and so I really related to what he said in his book. A program that would help the handicapped child's self-esteem would be worth it. The handicapped child has an even greater chance of experiencing low self-esteem since being "normal" in appearance and intelligence is the desired goal.

Up to this point, the room had been quiet as we listened politely. Then Chris said, "I'm going to change the mood of this room. You all look so inhibited!"

We watched her as she reached down and picked up a small drum. "My pupils enjoy playing the various instruments, and tonight I thought you might like to play them, too. It will loosen you up." The crowd moaned. "It's not going to be that awful; in fact, you might find yourself enjoying this."

I doubted that! I didn't want to make a fool of myself in this crowd. I was thinking of not playing the instrument when my turn came.

"Now I am going to lay out some rules. You have to play the instrument when it gets to you, and you cannot pass it until you have played it. Really—I know some of you do not want to do this—but do give it a try, and I promise you that you will enjoy it. For instruments that you probably do not know how to play, I will give a quick demonstration before giving them to you."

She passed the drum to the first person in the audience—we could hear a couple of faint beats on it. I was glad that I did not have to be the first person. He passed it on, and every few seconds we could hear another person banging on it. On and on Chris put instruments into the audience until an array of odd noises could be heard.

The first instrument reached Don, and he played it and handed it to me. It would have been so tempting to pass it on—only one problem, the person beside me was watching me! I felt foolish, but I did beat on the drum.

An odd thing happened when everyone had played a few instruments. People were laughing, and the instrument playing was getting more robust than at first. As much as I hated to admit it, it was fun. The crowd was talking and laughing. "This one is fun to play," the person next to Don said as he handed one instrument to him.

Chris was right—we were enjoying this, and the crowd was no longer inhibited. If she could spark a crowd of straightlaced people, what could she do with our special children?

Don and I went home, commenting that this had been an interesting and unusual evening!

Lessons I Needed to Learn

> And not only this, but we also exult in our tribulations,
> knowing that tribulation brings about perseverance; and
> perseverance, proven character; and proven character,
> hope; and hope does not disappoint, because the love of
> God has been poured out within our hearts through the
> Holy Spirit who was given to us (Rom. 5:3–5).

Lorie's music therapy began in March when she was
fourteen months old. She was a passive baby and the
youngest one Chris had ever worked with. The class
was a small one—Lorie and two little boys who were
about six months older than she.

Chris signaled the start of therapy time by spreading
a small, blue throw rug on the floor on which she
wanted the three little ones to sit. Lorie was the only
one who was faithful about staying on the rug and only
because she was not yet mobile. The little boys often
tried to wander off, but Chris was diligent about putting them back on the rug. Gradually, they got the idea
they were to stay put.

We mothers sat in on the sessions. This came about because one of the little boys would not cooperate unless his mother was nearby. He was stubborn, but eventually, Chris was able to get him to participate.

Looking back at it, I can see that *our watching the therapy sessions was a big mistake!* I was to learn a hard lesson from it.

Chris started her twice-weekly sessions with a song she called "Good Morning." She held each child, one at a time, on her lap and sang this song, which included his name. We mothers sang along, too.

This song seemed to loosen everyone up and gave Chris a chance to say a personal "hello" to the children.

From this point on, her program varied from session to session, as she determined how the little ones were learning and progressing. If their attention dwindled, she would turn to a more lively activity. If they seemed to be concentrating, she would teach them a new task or do one of the harder items.

Another song was "I Like." It was flexible in that Chris could add many words to go with "I Like:" I like Lorie; I like Mommy; I like cookies. Chris hoped this little song would teach them new words.

Chris taught them hand motions to go with rhymes, such as "Insey Tinsey Spider," "Wheels on the Bus," "Hickory Dickory Dock," and so on. The first one that Lorie learned the hand motions to was "Hickory Dickory Dock."

"Put Your Finger On" was a song that could be used with naming and touching their noses, shoes, or whatever Chris decided to name.

We mothers were not allowed to help our children put their fingers on what Chris said. She would name the object, and she herself would point to it. She wanted the little ones to copy her and do it on their own.

Chris worked at teaching them how to play some of the easier instruments. Some of the instruments and what the child learns from playing each are listed in the following chart.

Instrument	How Played	Skills	Variations
Songbells	Played with mallets	Eye-hand coordination	With or without music
		Reinforce letter reading	Stressing visual or auditory skills
		Improving visual dis-crimination	Hands together or separate
		Improving auditory dis-crimination	
		Visual tracking	
		Fine motor coordination	
Drum and rhythm instru-ments	Hit with two sticks; hit together or shake	Coordination, rhythm	Learning to follow drum notation or playing by listening
		Two hands steadily together	Playing at varied volumes to express feelings
		Following an auditory cue, or	
		Following a visual cue Emotional release	

Lorie

The songbells looked like a small piano keyboard, and Lorie liked to play this one. She would bang with her stick, and every once in awhile she would hit a key. Chris did not write letters on the keys but put colored marks on them instead. She would try to get them to play the key with the color she named and pointed at, for instance, the key with the red mark.

Chris worked with them on a little game with three ice-cream buckets filled with scraps of material. She would show the children an instrument, and then before their eyes, hide it in with the scraps of material. She wanted them to find the instrument. Lorie would start to look, but she would soon forget what she was looking for. Besides, she thought it was more fun to play with the pretty scraps of material.

As time went on, Chris tried new games and dropped old ones, but she kept the half-hour sessions busy ones! I marveled at how easy it was for Chris to work with the children—there was no doubt she loved them.

At first, I had really enjoyed watching the sessions. It was exciting, and I was learning from it; but one day it changed. I really didn't know what the problem was— there just seemed to be tension among us moms. We didn't seem to be visiting as freely as we had before. Oh, there wasn't any fighting or nasty remarks. But I noticed that my attitude was really ugly when I was there. The Lord was starting to show me something I really did not want to see! There was competitiveness among us mothers concerning our little ones. I wanted Lorie to be better than the others. In fact, I wanted her to be the best. I would watch, and if Lorie did something the other two didn't, I'd gloat! I certainly wasn't humble in this situation! If Lorie did poorly that day, I would tell everyone that she was probably starting to teethe, or maybe she was coming down with a cold.

I didn't realize what I was doing for quite awhile. It was under the surface and kept growing, until one day it had mushroomed into something big and ugly! Then I couldn't help but see it!

I really didn't want the boys to do as well as Lorie, and I could sense the other mothers felt this way too concerning their child. The unspoken undercurrent among the mothers was, "Mine did it; yours didn't!"

I was just starting to realize this when the two little boys left the music therapy program to enter the Day Activity Center.

As I came to terms with the problem and talked to a few people I trusted, I was able to get the thing in perspective. I was utterly ashamed of how I had acted! When Kevin was a baby, I had been competitive, and somehow, I hadn't learned my lesson then.

I began the healing process by first acknowledging to God my wrong attitude—oh, Lord, how wrong I had been! The other day I talked with one of the mothers, and we had such a nice visit! We were genuinely happy for what each other's child was doing, and I did not compare Lorie with her son. I saw the children as two distinct individuals developing in the way God has planned for them. What an important lesson I had learned!

Down's parents can be highly competitive. It's easy to compare our children when we are at therapy sessions, at coffees, or in parents' groups. Nothing is wrong with talking about our children or being happy when they do something new. The problem is when we compare, are jealous and competitive, or let other problems enter the picture.

During this time, I was also to learn another lesson. It came about with Lorie's sixteen-month developmental assessment, and this was the first time she would be tested on the Bayley scales of mental and motor development.

I had heard so much about how the Bayley scales differed from the Uzgiris-Hunt scales. Lorie had been tested on the Uzgiris-Hunt scale three times, at five, nine, and thirteen months. She had done fairly well on these.

Some of my friends' children who were older than Lorie had already been tested on the Bayley test, and they told me their children had done well. I became apprehensive and didn't look forward to the time when the "Laugh and Smile" people would test Lorie. With Lorie being slower physically and so passive and non-motivated, I felt she would not do well. And I didn't want to tell others if Lorie did poorly, especially my friends whose children had tested so well!

The day Dante arrived to administer the test, I was uptight during the whole time of testing. Dante started putting out some of the paraphernalia he had brought for the testing, while I put Lorie in her high chair. I took a seat at the table and watched nervously as he started the test.

The first thing Dante tested Lorie on was a red puzzle board with three geometrical designs, a circle, square, and triangle. He wanted Lorie to put the shapes in the correct spot. Lorie fiddled with this and did get the circle in its proper space.

Dante continued his testing while I sat on the edge of my chair. Some of the testing involved following a verbal command, such as "Put dolly in the chair . . . wipe dolly's face . . . put pegs in the holes . . . stack blocks . . . turn pages of the book . . . squeak the whistle doll," and many other items. Each time he would mark down how she did.

When the test was completed, Dante did not tell me

anything, whether Lorie had done well, poorly, or just adequately. He really didn't need to, as I had read his reactions and knew that Lorie hadn't done as well as he had expected. Disappointment welled up inside me. I tried to tell myself it didn't matter, but *it did matter!*

I became depressed for several days. I later learned from reading Tim LaHaye's book *How to Win Over Depression* that depression comes from a negative thinking pattern—you think yourself into it! Depression is anger frozen inside.

My disappointment had led to my being angry, hurt, and feeling sorry for myself. I was angry that Lorie had done poorly on the test! I had faced the fact that she was one of the slower ones in her physical development, and now I would have to face the fact that she might be one of the slower ones in the area of mental development. How much more could I take?

"Jesus, what are You trying to teach me? What do I need to learn?"

I was going through this at the same time that I was coming to terms with my ugly attitude at music therapy. I was to learn much the same thing in both of these situations. I had to accept Lorie as she was—physically, mentally, active or passive—and give up *all* my undue expectations. With those out of the way, I would have to do what was best for Lorie, not me, and try to give her the best preparation for the future.

Lorie was growing nicely and her check-ups were good health-wise. It was something to be thankful about. Her fifteen-month check-up weighed her in at seventeen pounds six ounces, and she was twenty-seven inches long.

Lorie was coming along in her physical development and was building up her list of accomplishments. At fifteen months she learned how to get from a sitting position to her stomach. Her seventeen-month accomplishments were learning how to get up and into a sitting position by herself and how to belly crawl.

When Lorie was nineteen months old, Kevin saw her pull herself up to a standing position at the bathtub. Lorie started crawling on her hands and knees at twenty-one months, something we didn't know if she would ever do because she has a loose hip problem. (She was so loose that she could do the splits without any problem at all. When she first learned how to sit up, she did the splits, and pulled herself up. You should have seen the reactions that caused! People were always asking, "How can she do that?")

After the boys left music therapy, Chris continued working with Lorie alone. This turned out to be good—the hours of individual stimulation helped Lorie become less passive.

Now therapy was held at Chris's house, and Chris worked with Lorie upstairs in a spare bedroom. I no longer watched the therapy sessions, and I liked this arrangement a lot better. If Lorie did something really neat, Chris would bring her down and have her show me. I loved being able to see the accomplished feat, and Lorie loved to show off to her mommy.

Don and I were excited with how much music therapy seemed to be helping Lorie. We were seeing Lorie emerge from a cocoon. Lorie was becoming like a beautiful butterfly; we were seeing so many, many lovely things in her. We learned that she has a sparkling personality, and that she is a fighter who is willing to work to overcome many drawbacks.

Looking back, I can see that it was during this time period that the Lord taught me the most about adjusting to and accepting Lorie. How the lessons hurt at the time, but today I can say they were all for my own good.

Just as I had learned to accept Lorie where she was in her development, the Lord had new things He wanted me to learn. He wanted me to thank Him for giving us Lorie.

One night our minister taught from the Bible about how we are to give thanks to God in everything, not just the good situations, but everything!

I couldn't believe God wanted us to thank Him for the awful things in life! Why? I just couldn't understand!

The minister told us we might not be thankful for the situation, but it is God's will for us to thank God in everything. He told us that God gives us a peace to guard our hearts. God wants us to be anxious about nothing!

The Lord asked me again and again during the next few days if I could thank Him for Lorie. Could I accept her as His will for our lives? I thought about what our minister had taught us at the Friday-night Bible study.

About midweek, I decided to make the blind leap of faith and thank Him for Lorie. I really didn't understand why I should thank Him for a situation that I really wasn't thankful about. I was indeed doing this out of faith. I got down on my knees in our living room and thanked God for Lorie!

I had made a big step in my growth. Oh, nothing marked this big step; no band marched in front of our house; no announcement was made on the six o'clock news. In fact, the world continued as if nothing had happened. But I knew something had happened. Peace settled over me, and I felt the contentment of doing the Lord's will.

I had learned in that quiet moment with the Lord to thank Him for giving us Lorie, even though I didn't fully understand why. I have a long, long way to go in trusting the Lord in every area of my life, but at that moment He had taken me one step further when I thanked Him for Lorie.

Lorie

Lorie was tested again on the Uzgiris-Hunt test at nineteen months, and this time the results were different. Lorie had improved so much that Dante commented on how much better she had done this time. Don and I were both excited! We both felt music therapy had a lot to do with it, plus the fact that Lorie was becoming more and more active. Could her improvement be a sign she might continue to do better? I hardly dared to hope for fear I would be disappointed again!

Would You Believe
I Have a Jealousy Problem?

Blessed be the God and Father of our Lord Jesus Christ, the Father of mercies and God of all comfort; who comforts us in all our affliction so that we may be able to comfort those who are in any affliction with the comfort with which we ourselves are comforted by God. For just as the sufferings of Christ are ours in abundance, so also our comfort is abundant through Christ (2 Cor. 1:3–5).

Don and I were able to learn more about Lorie as our friendship with the "Laugh and Smile" research people grew.

Our getting to know Linda came about because she was the one who usually came out to administer the laughter items. She would come with another student in the project, and together they would have me do the list of items to see how Lorie would respond—laugh, smile, or cry. We saw Dante at every lab test, and he gave the Bayley tests to Lorie.

We often saw Linda and Dante at various parent

get-togethers, and when Dr. Poor's group was in process, Dante once came to speak to us.

One of the things we liked about the "Laugh and Smile" research people was that they took the time to get to know us as parents. Whenever they would see us, they would visit with us, and we could call them if we had a question or a problem.

"We like to help the parents," Dante told me one day. "The early months are trying times, and it helps to have an expert in your corner, not a person who makes you feel guilty or puts your child down."

Dante's reaching out to us through himself and his staff helped. There are many rough times while adjusting to and trying to learn what is involved with a Down's Syndrome child.

A young man in his twenties, Dante became interested in the field of mental retardation back in his early years, because his closest friend had a brother who was retarded.

"I realized the amount of information about the retarded is skimpy," Dante once told us. "My interest in Down's Syndrome children came because there is even less known about their development than about other mentally handicapped children.

"Most of what I read on this subject was based on myths or stereotyped ideas about Down's. I found these children interesting, and I discovered that I could learn a lot about them by comparing them to normal children. I can learn about the process of development by seeing what is similar in Down's and normal babies and by finding out where the differences lie."

Dante was twenty-two years old when he began his research program as a graduate student at the university working toward his doctorate in clinical psychology and child development. His research program began early in 1974 with the last child completing the

"Laugh and Smile" part of the research in December, 1976.

The part of the "Laugh and Smile" project involving Lorie was held in our home twice a month from the time she was four months old until she reached the age of two years. Lorie was one of the twenty-five Down's infants in the home study. The other "Laugh and Smile" group numbered sixty, and they were brought into the lab at the ages of four, eight, twelve, fifteen, sixteen, twenty, and twenty-four months. Dante had the Bayley and Uzgiris-Hunt tests administered to all the children who participated in either "Laugh and Smile" group.

Dante's testing did not end with the "Laughter" studies. He continued with lab tests such as Loom, Visual Cliff, Strange to Strange Situation, and a new test Lorie took recently with a moving box.

When Dante was twenty-five years old, he was the youngest person ever to present a paper at the Down's Syndrome Congress, which is attended by about five hundred people. The Down's Syndrome Congress is an organization that is part of the National Association for Retarded Citizens.

Dante presented his paper on his research program, telling the various things that were done and what some of the basic findings were. "We are finding out that the development of these babies is similar to that of normal babies," he told the congress.

Because Lorie had been so much slower in her physical development than some other Down's Syndrome children, I was interested in what Dante had to say concerning her development.

"Parents should be aware that most lay people equate motor development with intelligence in infancy. Basically, these ideas come out of books that show the development of locomotor milestones such as

123

crawling, walking, and so forth. A Down's baby can do well mentally, but be slow in his physical development, and this can fool you."

His words were a great help to me when I was struggling with Lorie in her physical development and learning the lessons the Lord was teaching me. Dante was a professional in our corner!

"It's important," Dante said, "that people who do research with handicapped children really be in it for the children. We have gotten close to the families, and in turn, we have learned a lot."

When Lorie started crawling, Dante had us bring her into the lab to do a test called the Visual Cliff. On one side it looked as if she was on solid ground (the "shallow" side), and on the other side it looked as if she would fall off the edge (the "deep" side). A large piece of plexiglass covered the whole area so that Lorie would not fall.

The test was run four times, two times with Lorie on the "shallow" side and two times on the "deep" edge; this measured depth perception.

I stood on the opposite side and tried to coax Lorie to come to me. When Lorie was first placed on the "shallow" side, she did not come onto the "deep" edge, even though I had tried to coax her in every way I could think of. When placed on the "deep" edge, Lorie sprawled out and peered at the area below her. She did not like this and crawled off to the safety of the "shallow" side. Afterward, Dante told us that she had done what he wanted her to do.

At nineteen months, Lorie was tested for the first time in a test called the Strange Situation. This test started when Lorie and I entered an empty room where I placed her on the floor to play with the toys that they had put out for her. Lorie started to play contentedly with them while I watched from a nearby chair.

Would You Believe I Have a Jealousy Problem?

Dante had a time sequence planned with things he wanted to do to conduct this experiment. First, Lorie and I were alone in a room; then a stranger joined us, but we were not to talk. Next the stranger and I visited; the stranger and Lorie played; I left Lorie with the stranger and returned; Lorie was left alone; the stranger reentered; and finally I returned.

Dante wanted to see how Lorie would react in each situation. Would she continue to play when I left? Would she look for me? Would she cry, or act as if she didn't miss me?

Afterward we were able to view the whole testing sequence on videotape. Lorie did not cry or look for me after I left the room, nor did the stranger bother her. She simply continued playing. When she was older, she was tested again. The second time, she cried and looked for me. This meant that she was beginning to become her own person and express her feelings.

The main hope Don and I had, when we consented to Lorie's being in the research program, is that Dante's research findings would help make a difference for the Down's Syndrome person in the areas of being understood by others, educational programs, and the kind of life they can have as adults.

Cris, my neighbor not the music therapist, became a good friend of mine in the summer months. We had many things in common—the same age, married the same number of years, and two children, a boy and a girl. Also we had both received professional help for mental depression—I many years before she.

Cris and I shared our ups and downs, our victories and failures, and knew that we could depend on each other. We read the same Christian books and often discussed what we had learned from them and how they had helped us.

I have learned, and still am learning, many things

from Cris. One morning, after we had finished discussing a recent book, our conversation changed to some of the new things that Cris had been learning.

Cris said, "One thing is that in every situation you have a choice. You can complain, whine, blame someone else, or turn it around and see what you can learn from it."

This was a new concept for me, and I kicked it around in my mind the next few days. Could I adapt this idea to go along with the Scripture verse that tells us to give God thanks in *everything*?

It wasn't too long afterward that the Lord started using small irritations in my life to put this idea into use.

When I spilled a glass of milk on the floor, instead of overreacting, I thanked God and tried to determine what I could learn from it. A few days and several more minor irritations later, followed by giving thanks, I was starting to see something. Minor irritations weren't bothering me as much as they used to, and I was able to handle them without getting upset, depressed, or feeling the world was against me. My patience was improving! I was excited to learn that things that used to bother me were not bothering me in the same way. Turning a normally frustrating situation around, I was able to see that God was teaching me to respond better.

One day I applied this concept to our receiving Lorie. I was trying to see how many ways I could find to turn this around. I don't often complain to other people about all the extra things involved with Lorie, but I do let my mind run races around the negative factors, and often, this makes me depressed.

I have constructed a mental list, a list that I recall when I need some positive feedback:

• Lorie is helping me to understand about mentally retarded people in a different way than I had previously. I can remember that when I was in school and saw the mentally retarded students, I was thankful I was not one of the "dumb" students. I had gone through years of thinking I was better than they. The Lord has brought a little daughter into my life to teach me otherwise.

• I have learned how to reach out to others since Lorie came into my life. I am more understanding of my friends and family when problems and hard times enter their lives. I am more concerned about other people.

• Lorie was and still is the tool the Lord is using in our lives to bring us to Him.

• It helps me to have to put Lorie first and myself second throughout most of the week. I am busy taking her to therapy sessions and working with her when we are at home. It is making me become more of a serving person. I really have to put out to give her the best possible start in life.

• Lorie has indirectly brought people to the Lord.

• Lorie is a beautiful example to the world of what handicapped children can do. These children are really overcomers! Lorie has been an amazement to many people who, knowing so little about Down's Syndrome, are surprised when they discover she isn't anything like they thought she would be.

• Lorie has taught me to give thanks to God in everything, even though many times I haven't always felt thankful.

• Having a special child has given me an interest in trying to show the public a more positive concept of what a Down's person is really like. I would like people to see the Down's individual as a person and not as someone who is different; to see that he is an over-comer and can be a useful person with our help.

● I have learned to quit focusing on the negative things and to thank God for the many good things instead. I am thankful to God that Lorie is one of the healthiest Down's Syndrome children we know! My giving thanks has reached out to different areas of our lives—for Don's job, our nice home, our large garden; for the early intervention and continuing programs for Lorie to help her make it in this world; and for the gift of our normal son.

● I thanked God for using Lorie to reach us and bring us to Him.

My list could go on and on. Many times I add a new item to think about. The more I think about the positive factors of receiving Lorie, the more I realize how differ-ent my attitude has become. I no longer feel sorry about having her; I no longer wish she were normal or feel that rearing her is a lot of work and a long struggle. I wouldn't trade her for the world! As I have been able to view my situation with a thankful and positive attitude in others. Lorie is reflecting a good image by her own little outgoing personality, her ability to be an over-comer and her own unique individuality. She is cer-tainly different than the stereotype that the world be-lieves about Down's Syndrome people.

I have learned to use this turning-around process in other areas of my life where God is working to teach me a lesson, as I know He will all the rest of my life.

A few months ago I was told that I had a bitterness problem, and believe me, it hurt when I was told! The first few days I felt hurt and angry, and I really didn't want to admit to anyone that I had this problem. I was able to confide only in Don and Cris about it.

Then shortly afterward, I sat down and thanked God for showing me this area and started turning this situation around.

I listed the negative and positive factors and thought about them for several days. I had been hurt by the fact that the person who saw the bitterness in me told Don and not me! I could not change this fact, but I could thank God that He had used this way to show the problem to me. And knowing this, I could let Him change me.

As I faced my feelings, both negative and positive, I was able to understand what had been causing my bitterness and to let God work through me in this situation.

Slowly, but surely, the Lord is changing many of Don's and my attitudes and outlooks concerning Lorie and what we show the world about her. Today a girl friend told me, "You used to be negative about Lorie, and it came across that you thought of Lorie as less than a person. You have changed, and the last time we saw you, we really noticed it. Now you act as if Lorie is like any other child; sure, she is different, but that doesn't seem to matter to you—you love her anyway!"

I now know that to get us from step A to B, C, D, and so on, God uses many situations, and though they hurt at the time, eventually we thank God for them. These teaching situations have helped me become what I am today in accepting Lorie and mirroring this. I'm sure there are many other lessons up the road, and I know God will use them to teach me even more.

One big lesson I learned began on a hot, July evening when we were at Sunday church services. The big news of the evening was that one of the couples had had their third normal boy the day before. Everyone was happy about it except me! I was ashamed of how I was feeling and reacting, but I couldn't seem to control it. Negative feelings welled up inside of me, and I kept trying to stuff them down.

Stan, the proud papa, strolled in and was greeted by several people.

"How are Pat and the baby?" one person asked.

"Fine, just fine," Stan answered in his easy, carefree manner.

"Gee, we didn't think you would be here!" another person commented.

Stan was every bit the proud dad telling everyone his new son's birth weight and what they had named him. He showed everyone the Polaroid picture he had snapped of his new son.

Tears crept to the edge of my eyes, and I tried to brush them away. I was trying so hard to keep my jumble of feelings and emotions under control. It was like fighting a major battle in my mind, and right then I was almost losing.

The night became a blur as I tried not to face the real feelings and thoughts that tried to rise to the surface. At this time, I did not know much about dealing with both negative and positive feelings in a constructive way.

Thoughts ran through my mind—a continual attack —and some of them were: *We only wanted to have two normal children. Why couldn't we have this? Why did they get three normal babies? Everything works out for other people and not for us!* I was really in a self-pity bag (as Cris calls it) and very jealous! I wanted to get up and scream: *It's not fair! It's not fair!*

It's funny how we can act as if we have everything under control—that we are *such nice* people—but yet, if people could see us on the inside, they would see something else. That night they would have seen a very ugly person inside me!

When we got into the car to go home, everything burst out. I could no longer control it, and the battle that had been raging inside me won. I screamed, yelled, and complained to Don, and caused him to become angry. I knew what I was doing, yet somehow, I couldn't stop myself.

When we arrived home, Don had to shake me to get me to come to my senses. Then guilt, shame, and sorrow erupted from within me, and I cried a lot. I was so ashamed of how I had acted that I wanted to disappear through the nearest crack!

The next day I still didn't like myself. I hated how I had acted the night before and was ashamed of how I had reacted to Stan and Pat's new son. I certainly did not wish a handicapped child on them just because we had one.

I told Jesus how ashamed I was; I asked Don's forgiveness, and I knew that God had to work on my horrible jealousy problem.

Coming to terms with jealousy did not happen overnight, but slowly I began to turn this around and learn how and why I had reacted the way I had.

As time has passed, jealousy has faded into the background, and I can be genuinely happy when a baby arrives and is normal. To reach this stage of acceptance, I had to come to terms with the fact that I was jealous! God had to open this door, even though I wanted to keep the door shut.

September arrived, and with it, my folks for a week-long visit. The night before Lorie's next music therapy session, Chris called. "Mary Ann, dress Lorie in something nice for tomorrow's session."

"Why?" I asked curiously.

"Would you believe the *Tribune* is going to interview me for a write-up in one of their columns?"

"Really? How neat!" I was excited; what a great chance to show a positive picture about handicapped children.

"And," Chris continued, "we are going to use my working with Lorie as the picture for the feature!"

I hung up the phone and told my parents that something really exciting was going to happen during their visit.

Tomorrow was going to be a big day!

People, Not God, Put Labels on People

So that all the peoples of the earth may know that the
Lord is God; there is no one else (1 Kings 8:60).

A few days after the interview had taken place, the
phone rang early one morning.

"Mary Ann," Chris's excited voice came across the
telephone lines, "the article is in today's paper, and it is
super! Here, let me read you some parts from it!"

I listened, and oh, how anxious this made me to buy
a newspaper so that I could see the column!

"And," Chris continued, "the article is all positive.
I'm so happy with the way the reporter has written it!"

Caught up in Chris's excitement, I told her, "I can
hardly wait to see it! What does Lorie's picture look
like?"

"It's just darling. They picked a cute pose of her, and
it looks natural. I'm sure you will like the article as well
as I do."

It wasn't too long after Kevin had left on the school

bus that Mom, Dad, Lorie, and I were off to the store.

Back in Dad's car, with several copies of the paper, I tore through one of the copies to find the column. I began to read it and to admire Lorie and Chris's picture.

There wasn't a doubt that I was excited about the positive nature of the article! It was and still is my dream to show the public a positive picture of the Down's Syndrome person. How good it was that Lorie could help show the public some of the positive factors of special children and the programs that could help them. Lorie was able to be a star by just being herself!

Recently, Chris and I were talking about the newspaper article. "How did the newspaper hear about you and set up the interview?" I asked her as we were enjoying a glass of iced tea together.

"I really don't know. Maybe it was from the other newspapers who have written about me and my work." About the man who interviewed her, Chris said, "It was interesting that he was normally a sports reporter. When he arrived for the interview, he did not see the implications of Lorie's being retarded. This is how I wanted him to see Lorie! He really was a fantastic person. I liked him and was pleased with the way he wrote the article.

She continued, "He made it seem as if Lorie was a normal child. When describing Lorie, he just described a child! This way it gives the public the idea that Lorie is not different. You do not want people to set her aside as being different. When people comment, 'She can do that?' you say, 'Of course, she can do that!' If the average person can accept that these children can do things like normal children (just slower), it will make a big difference in their acceptance in the world.

"I don't think," Chris said, "the outside world really needs to know all that is involved with getting your child to the point where she is. Just as in the case of a good singer, you never know how hard he or she worked to reach this degree of excellence. You want them to see the story and not dwell on all the hard work that is involved. You want them to see the wonderful person that Lorie is and all the things she can do!"

"What were some of the comments you heard after the newspaper article came out?" I asked Chris.

"Some of the people, after reading the article, commented, 'What is so unusual about what Lorie can do? Any baby can do these things.' They did not see Lorie as being handicapped or different."

My mind was mulling over that thought. Wouldn't this be a neat concept—to show the world that these children are not so different or strange and that they act and function similarly to the normal child?

"Most of the comments I heard," I told Chris, "were how well they thought the article had been written and how positive it sounded."

There is no doubt we have to get across to the public that these children are people, that they think and have feelings and emotions, and that, with our help they can be useful people. *We must see them as individuals and not as something different!*

Chris had been instrumental in teaching me the lesson of seeing Lorie as a person and not as someone who is "different." I carried the concept of Lorie's being different from my past teachings of mental retardation.

It's funny, as I look back to the time when I learned this lesson, that I even felt, thought, and responded the way I did. This was the last of the big lessons the Lord was to teach me in working toward the goal of full acceptance of Lorie as God had made her.

To me, Lorie did not seem to carry as many Down's features as some of the other Down's children I know. And to me, if she didn't look like a Down's child, then people wouldn't really know. I often commented to Chris how happy I was that Lorie did not look much like a Down's child—maybe she really did, but I wanted to convince myself that she didn't. The issue, to Chris, was not how Lorie looked, but that Lorie be considered a person.

One day, after I had made the same comment (I must have sounded like a broken record!), Chris intervened. "You know, God didn't put the label of handicapped on Lorie. People did, and their labels dictate what is considered to be *normal* and *not normal.*"

Chris' statement stunned me, and I stopped in my tracks to think over what she had told me. In fact, I spent many days thinking about it. What she had said made me do a lot of thinking on exactly what my concept of Lorie was. I always seemed to be emphasizing the fact that Lorie was Down's Syndrome (different) and never seeing her just as a person.

It was true. I had to change my thinking. Lorie is a person, a very special person, and my daughter, whom I love.

To begin the turning-around process, I had to agree with God that I saw this problem, thank Him, and ask for a new attitude.

Today, the results of the change are reflected in my current attitudes concerning handicapped people. Now I realize they have feelings, emotions, goals, dreams, and aspirations—just like us! Their goals may be somewhat different in context than ours, but they have them! I do not think of Lorie as being unusual anymore; I just see her as our daughter and a person in her own right.

Coming back to my recent visit with Chris, our conversation continued and I told her how much her statement had helped me in coming to terms with the fact that Lorie is a person!

People, Not God, Put Labels on People

Chris said, "God didn't make handicapped children; He just made them differently. In fact, many people we call handicapped today would not have been labeled such a hundred years ago.

"There is nothing wrong with Lorie the way she is," Chris continued. "This is a wrong concept that parents have today. If Lorie is wrong, then you are saying you are right because you were born 'normal,' and this isn't so. People aren't made right or wrong; they are made people. By saying there is nothing wrong with the way Lorie is, we can then say that she is made differently and has a harder time in this world."

How much sense this statement made! The world did seem to consider a person born normal as right and the handicapped person as wrong! But what really is normal?

"When you used to say, 'Lorie doesn't look very Down's,' it was like saying a black person is not very black. It really doesn't make that much difference."

"That's true," I agreed. "A black person is black no matter what the shade of his skin."

Chris said, "When you would comment on wondering how people would respond to Lorie, especially as she got older, I would pick her up and wonder how anyone couldn't like her. She didn't seem any different; she was a little baby who was very lovable. Parents today can't worry now about the tomorrows and the things they may bring. You must just consider your child now and realize that he or she needs your love, reassurance, and guidance.

"Why do you need assurance that she is going to college or whatever? These are the types of goals you put on a normal two-year-old and don't even realize it—until you have a handicapped child who may not be able to accomplish some of your goals. To me, it is an advantage for parents to rear a special child."

137

I will always be grateful to Chris for being that professional friend who cared enough to help me work through my problems. She was in Lorie's and my life when we needed her, and for this, we will always be thankful.

Our Christian friends had once told Don and I that we may have a special ministry for Christ because of our daughter. During the summer months, we started to see this come about, first with a girl friend, and then with my sister and her husband.

Pat, a friend from Rochester, had called me one afternoon toward the end of May. She wanted Don to pick her up at the bus depot during a short layover; she was on her way home. I sensed something was wrong, and felt led to share Jesus with her.

I waited all the rest of the day and on into the evening in nervous anticipation. What was wrong? Why did she want to see us? Was she having marital problems?

It was a confused, mixed-up Pat whom I greeted at the door. My mind raced back to the first time I had seen her—it was just after we had moved to Rochester. An attractive, tall woman who knew how to dress well, Pat had once been a model. We met when we both worked at a bakery. She stayed one day and quit, while I braved it a couple of weeks and then left. We became friends, even though we were very much opposites!

Tonight Pat looked worn out, down in her spirits, and glad to see us again.

"I don't know why I had to see you, except that during the whole trip back, one thought kept running across my mind: 'Go see Don and Mary Ann!' This is all I have wanted to do since I left California."

"Is your problem your marriage?" I asked.

"Yes, and I don't want to fail again."

What a crazy night we spent. Don and I talked to her for quite awhile. She was indeed having problems in her marriage. She was broke and had only enough money to buy a bus ticket to get home, as her husband wasn't supporting her. She was going to her parents' home, because she had inherited some money from an aunt and was going home to get this taken care of.

Pat was confused about what to do with her failing marriage and glad to have time to think things over. "If he wants me and is willing to work at it, I will go back. I don't want a divorce!"

The conversation moved to spiritual things, and Pat really listened. In fact, she didn't want me to quit talking, and we stayed up all night.

We had wanted Pat to stay with us for a few days, but since she couldn't use the ticket another day, she decided to go on home. Her few hours here had certainly been packed ones!

I watched her ride off with Don in the morning and hoped that something I had told her about the Lord had sunk in. Something dawned on me that morning: the Lord had used our having Lorie, and what this had done in our lives, as a witness to Pat. We had been told we might have a ministry because of Lorie, and it was true. I told Pat about the Lord, and how He had used Lorie in our lives. The Lord showed us another reason why He gave us Lorie.

In July, a letter came from Pat, a sad letter that surprised us. Pat had planned to go back to her husband on the eighth, as all the legal papers were finally being completed on her inheritance. The morning of the fourth, she received a phone call saying that her husband had been killed in a motorcycle accident. Suddenly, she was a widow trying to cope with this sad news and getting ready to fly to his parents' home to make the funeral arrangements.

I quickly wrote her a letter to express our sorrow. As I was writing it, I felt impressed to tell her that her husband, who had not accepted the Lord, was lost, and she would be, too, if she didn't accept Jesus.

After I mailed the letter, I wondered if this would be the last I would hear from her. How would a grieving widow react to what I had said?

A few days later she phoned to say that after she read that paragraph, she asked Jesus into her heart. I was stunned! I was starting to learn that God can work through anything, and His way may be foreign to our thinking.

Pat couldn't understand why she was a widow, why her dreams of a good marriage and children had never come about. She understood only that Jesus had called her, and that she had accepted His invitation. Jesus used her sad situation to reach her, as He does with so many of us. A lot of us wouldn't accept Jesus if He didn't throw impossible situations in front of us.

(This February, 1978, we received a phone call; our friend Pat, who was twenty-nine, had passed away. Don and I were shocked, and tears rolled down my cheeks. I thanked God for bringing her to us and using us in her life. How comforting it is to know that she knew Him before He called her home.)

In August, my sister told me that Dale Evans was coming to speak in their town sometime in the fall. I wanted to go, especially since Dale Evans had been the parent of a Down's Syndrome daughter, too.

Don and I prayed to the Lord to see if He would provide the extra money for us to go. He did, and we went to my sister's home one weekend in October.

Peg and Bruce accompanied us, and we drove that lovely fall evening to the place where Dale Evans was to speak. We could sense the excitement in the audience. I wondered what she would talk about. Would she mention something about her Down's daughter, Robin, whose life they had shared for two years?

People, Not God, Put Labels on People

When Dale Evans came down the aisle and went up onto the stage, I strained to get a glimpse of her. She certainly was an attractive woman. She had a pleasant smile, and she greeted everyone with a warm and friendly voice. You could see the happiness of Jesus radiating from her.

The next few minutes passed quickly as she shared with us many parts of her life, including incidents concerning Robin. It was a beautiful talk that brought tears to my eyes.

At the end, she called people to come forward and ask Jesus to come into their lives if they were not in Him already and to ask Him to forgive their sins. Several people started down the aisle to give their lives to Jesus, and before our very eyes, we saw my sister, Peggy, and her husband, Bruce, make the trip down the aisle. They had heard Jesus calling them, and had gone forward.

I wanted to meet Dale Evans. Maybe it was a silly idea; after all, she certainly could not talk personally to everyone! But I wanted to tell her that we have a Down's Syndrome daughter. And I wanted her to know I had enjoyed reading about her and Roy Rogers in a book titled *The Answer is God* by Ellise Miller Davis. I had also read Dale Evans' book, *Angel Unaware*.

Don and I went toward the stage to see if we could get a couple of words with her, only to find that she had already left and that other people were tending to the people who had come forward. My feelings ranged from disappointment to sorrow, but surprisingly enough, I thanked God right away and accepted my not meeting her as His will for me.

Don decided to drive out by the airport to see if we could get a glimpse of her. We arrived just as her plane was flying off. A peace had filled my heart, and though I didn't get to meet her in person, I did get to hear her talk, and for this I was thankful!

"Are you disappointed?" my sister asked.

"No, not now. I was at first, but I realize that the Lord said 'no' to this desire."

We decided that we would stop at a nearby restaurant to have a treat and talk before we headed home to the children.

As we were driving to the place Bruce had suggested, a thought flashed across my mind: "Here you were so disappointed about not meeting Dale Evans in person that you missed the miracle. It started with wanting to see Dale Evans, and Peg and Bruce had come along. Didn't you see them go forward and and accept Jesus?"

I was ashamed. I had, indeed, been focusing on myself and not rejoicing in what the Lord had accomplished in my sister's and her husband's lives. God had brought them to Him, and this night of their accepting Him had started last February when I began to share Jesus with them. Dale Evans' talk had caused Peg to want to give her whole life to Jesus, and Bruce realized for the first time that the Lord is the answer to life's questions.

"Oh, Lord," I silently prayed, "thank You for reaching them. You never cease to amaze me!" I marveled at how God had used this situation. It had given Don and me a chance to see what had come from Dale Evans' life as a spinoff from the birth of her Down's Syndrome daughter. What had seemed a tragedy had been turned around to glorify Jesus Christ. And He reached out and added Bruce and Peggy to His family.

It's so exciting to see how God works in the lives of new Christians. We saw many changes in the early weeks with Peg and Bruce; they were different each time we saw them. The excitement of being in the Lord bubbled through their letters to us, and Don and I rejoiced in the things the Lord was doing in their lives.

One afternoon when my Christian girl friend, Joy, came over for a visit, she asked me, "Did you ever ask Jesus to heal Lorie?"

"No, this was the one thing Don and I never did."

"Why not?" Joy asked.

I sat for a couple of moments trying to compose my thoughts, and then I tried to tell her why we had never prayed this prayer. "At first, it never really dawned on me to request this, even after I had accepted the Lord. Later, as I grew in the Lord, I began to understand more and more that this was His will for our lives. He could have, when I was carrying Lorie, interceded, and made Lorie perfect, but He chose not to do so. The more that I realized this was His will for our lives, the more I knew that asking Him this would be saying that I did not want to accept receiving Lorie, a special child, as His will for our lives."

I could see Joy trying to understand what I was trying to tell her. She seemed a bit confused as I tried to explain our thoughts in this. "Are you saying other parents of handicapped children shouldn't pray for their children to be healed?"

"No, they have to do what they feel is right for them in their situation and what they know is God's will for them. One of my friends prayed for a healing of her daughter, and there is nothing wrong with this. I realize that the Lord answers prayers for healing in many different ways, and not always in a complete physical healing. This concept I learned in Joyce Landorf's book *Mourning Song*. The little girl was not healed physically, but I'm sure their prayer was answered in some way. Maybe it was answered in their having more acceptance of their daughter and her handicap."

"I guess I had never thought of healing in those terms," Joy told me.

"The book *Joni*, by Joni Eareckson, helped me to realize that God can do more through Lorie the way she is than He could do if He healed her," I continued. "And how true this statement is. Lorie has brought us to the Lord, plus many others indirectly. She has taught and is teaching us so many things. We are growing as we are reaching out to her and trying to make the best possible life for her."

I paused for a moment and then went on. "One thing that I did pray for was that Lorie be the best that is possible for her. I said this prayer when I learned from the Bible that 'you have not because you ask not.' I know that it would be easier to have Lorie normal, but then she would probably not have the powerful message concerning the Lord that she has today. I thank God for her and have accepted her as His will for our lives."

Joy's facial expression seemed to mirror some understanding, and I finished with this last statement: "I now understand that God never gives us something that we can't handle. He knew when He gave us Lorie that we could handle it and that she was what was best for us. It doesn't matter if we understand the whole idea of it. *The important thing is that He understands!* By faith, Don and I have accepted Lorie's being handicapped as His will for our lives and her life."

I have often prayed, "Oh, Lord, we don't understand why, and what the future involves for us with Lorie, but we know that You are controlling the whole situation and are guiding us along. We are depending on You!"

A Time of Victories

In this you greatly rejoice, even though for a little while, if necessary, you have been distressed by various trials, that the proof of your faith, being more precious than gold which is perishable, even though tested by fire, may be found to result in praise and glory and honor at the revelation of Jesus Christ; and though you have not seen Him, . . . you greatly rejoice with joy inexpressible and full of glory (1 Pet. 1:6–8).

December arrived, and with it the approaching Christmas season. I began wondering how my reaction would be this year to the holiday season and to Lorie's second birthday. Would it be as awful as last year? Old thoughts ran across my mind as I relived parts of the depressing previous Christmas season. How I hoped this year's celebration would be a lot better!

True to his last year's promise (to go away), Don whisked us off in the car to spend the holiday with my sister and her family.

The opening of Lorie's gifts became a big occasion, as everyone gathered around and watched the three boys help Lorie unwrap them. They "oh-ed" and "ah-ed" as the gifts were revealed from under the brightly colored wrappings. Lorie loved being the center of attention. Her eyes sparkled, and she bubbled with excitement as she saw what each package was. One of her gifts was a doll that she immediately clutched in her arms—she had found a new friend.

The change of scenery for Lorie's second birthday did wonders. Our visit was a busy time of tending to four children, opening Christmas presents, preparing and serving the holiday meal, visiting, trying to keep the house in some kind of order, and going to church on Sunday. On our way home I realized I hadn't even thought about our Christmas of two years before. I was happy that time was indeed putting those events further in the past and that we were being healed from the wound these events had caused.

Lorie tipped the scales at eighteen pounds and was twenty-nine inches long. She didn't look like a two-year-old, but we were happy with her growth.

Her list of accomplishments was growing: At twenty-one months she started to feed herself with a spoon and sometimes managed to get some food into her mouth! At twenty-two months she was starting to stand alone for a few seconds at a time, and by the age of two, I was amazed at how many things she could say. She didn't seem interested in walking, but managed to get wherever she wanted to go by crawling. I never knew where I would find her or what she would be doing next.

Lorie's second birthday meant that she was eligible to enter the Day Activity Center, and she started in January. I drove her to school the first day, and from then on, she was bused to and from school. My feelings ran rampant that first day as I drove the car closer and closer to the school. I couldn't pinpoint which one of my feelings was predominate, but I was *tempted* to turn the car around and run back to the safety of home with my daughter! She seemed too small to be going to school.

We pulled up in front of the building, and I sat in the car a couple of minutes relishing the time with Lorie before we entered the building. This day marked a big change in our lives. Lorie would be going to school five days a week.

Lorie and I left the car and went the short distance to enter the building. Lorie was quickly taken from my arms; her snowsuit was removed, and she was placed in a large room with several other small children. Lorie was not crying as I walked out of the building and down the walk to my car. I felt empty. Still, I knew deep down that this was the best thing for her, and I had to overcome my selfish feelings of wanting to keep her at home with me. Lorie needed a good start in life, and this is why Don and I placed her in the Day Activity Center.

How tightly I hugged Lorie for the first few days after she arrived home from school! I really missed her during the day. After the first day, I wondered how she had done during the day. Thank heaven, her teacher knew I would have these questions, and she called to tell me how Lorie's first day had gone.

Now, Rae-ann, Lorie's teacher, sends a small notebook home with Lorie in which she writes of the things Lorie has done in school, and I write back things Lorie has done at home. These notes keep me posted on Lorie's accomplishments.

The first week of school, Lorie cried off and on at the more aggressive children, (they scared her), at being driven off in the school van, or at other things that seemed to bother her. By the end of the first week, she gave up crying and seemed to be enjoying going off to school. Nowadays, she waves me a happy good-bye. She likes school!

Lorie

A note Rae-ann sent me at the beginning of Lorie's schooling, dated January 6, 1977, reads: "Lorie had a good day. She cried when someone opened and closed our door; otherwise, she was fine. I think she'll feel more secure as times goes on. Sincerely, Rae-ann."

The first week of Lorie's going to school was harder on me than it was on her! Other than a few crying spells, she seemed to manage fine. I, on the other hand, fought mixed emotions, depression, emptiness, and trying to adjust to having free time. The previous two years had been hectic with all that was involved with Lorie, along with my other duties. The free time became enjoyable as time went on. With my morning work getting done faster, I had time to do some of the things I had not been able to do before.

Don and I are both happy to see Lorie's new accomplishments that have come from her special schooling. I get excited every time I see something new that she has learned. We are thankful for the people who are helping Lorie learn new things and guiding her along the rough road she has ahead of her.

And I am now being able to enjoy Lorie just as my daughter, and this is fun! The first two years were so busy I did not have much time to enjoy her. I was busy running her to therapy, exercising her, plus doing all the work that is involved with any baby. I now enjoy her and teach her things on my own, just as I did with her brother when he was her age.

I like watching her play and some of the antics she is now doing. If she sees me brushing my teeth, she often runs her fingers across her teeth—she is a great mimic! And if she sees me getting ready to go somewhere, her arms immediately go up, and she lets me know she doesn't want to be left behind! "Bye-bye, bye-bye!" she demands.

Lorie arrives home from school happy to see me and anxious to head off on some exploring. She throws the contents of drawers around; she scatters Kleenex around the house or strings toilet tissue in the bathroom. She is a climber and often pushes the step stool over to where she wants to be. One day I found her on the kitchen cupboard rattling my coffee mug tree around. Or she and the puppy play together and sometimes play too roughly. I hear one of them protesting and have to rush to the injured victim. In case you haven't guessed, Lorie is an active little girl and certainly not the passive child we were led to believe she would be in the beginning.

The following is a progress report of Lorie's schooling from various notes written by her teacher during the winter and summer sessions, 1977.

March 22—Lorie is doing more standing and walking activities every week. We march with our streamers around the table; usually she goes around once and then wants to sit down. Today she just kept right on walking around until the marching music stopped.

March 28—Lorie seemed to be watching the sound signals for different words much closer today. We are working on the "T" sound, and she seems to be placing her tongue in the correct position. We call it our clock sound because of the tick-tick of the clock. No "F" sound yet from her, but she watches my mouth closely. [The teacher uses sound signals in their program of helping these children learn how to talk.]

March 31—We fingerpainted today with shaving cream; Lorie thought this was really something. She patted it and smeared it and got it as far as her reach would allow.

Lorie

April 15—We went outside to play for the first time this spring. Lorie loved it! I took her down the slide with me and she got quite a look on her face. We also had a picnic lunch outside; we had hot dogs and other finger foods. Lorie would look up when she was eating to look at the birds, and she looked as if she wanted to say, "Boy, this is different."

April 19—Lorie walked three to four steps at different times again today. She seems pleased with herself, doesn't she? Today we worked on the "K" sound and she said "cake" quite clearly. Is that a new word or has she said it before?

April 26—I agree she is a climber! Out in the playroom, she tried climbing up the climber just like the big children. She sometimes seems to scold when she can't climb up as high as the boys.

April 27—We went outside to play today. As you can tell from Lorie's clothes, she played in the sandbox and enjoyed herself immensely. When we play our listening game, Lorie does so well. I say, "Who's listening?" and then tell one of the children to do a certain action, like "stamp your feet," "put your hands on your head." Lorie listens and does almost all the actions.

May 2—Lorie did the sound signal and said both the "K" and "B" words. She just seemed so happy to do it. Have you been using the sound signals at home?

She was looking at pictures and saw a dog and it sounded as if she said "dog" and then petted the picture of the dog. Very interesting about Lorie withholding at the "U" [Dante's research] something she could do, when we were just talking about her doing that on Friday.

A Time of Victories

May 4—We fingerpainted today and we could hardly get Lorie away from the table, as she was so involved. She insists on walking up the steps by herself now.

May 5—Today we listened to the Language Master and looked at the pictures. Lorie sat and listened and looked at them. She tried saying "cat" when she heard it on the L.M. and saw the picture.

She was really active today. We set up an obstacle course in the room. A little "mountain" to crawl over, a "tunnel" to crawl through, and "something" to step into. Lorie got right in and was climbing up, crawling through, and sliding down. I remember in January when she was overwhelmed by all the activity and would sit away from us and watch, but wouldn't join in. She joined in today!

May 9—Lorie walked six to eight steps to the door today and seemed very pleased with herself. She blew out our candle four times and would clap and giggle each time she did it.

May 13—We had a fun day—a birthday party plus playing outside. Lorie loved playing in the sandbox, but I'm afraid her outfit shows it. She plays around with the other children more and more and doesn't seem to feel threatened by their activity.

May 16—Lorie seemed hesitant to walk at all today. She stood fine for long periods of time, but she didn't take many steps. She did so much better putting the circle and square in the form board. She also blew the candle out several times and was forming her mouth well for the blowing. [Blowing is used for teaching pre-speech.]

Lorie

May 25—Lorie did more walking today than she has done lately, but she makes a game of it. But that's fine, because walking is supposed to be fun, right?

She listened to our story so well and did some of the actions along with me as I was telling the story.

June 17—It looks as if during the summer I'll probably get a note written on just Friday. The morning goes so fast, it's unbelievable. [Lorie goes half a day to summer school.]

Lorie seems happy to be back. She is doing actions to our songs and finger plays very well. On Wednesday, she walked five steps, let herself down, walked five more steps, and let herself back down, walked five more steps and let herself back down, and got up and walked another five steps.

She doesn't seem to like the young volunteers because they want to pick her up and cuddle her; she is getting to be "Little Miss Independent."

Oh, yesterday Lorie said "o" for open. We have a treat box with a lid on it and we say "open" each time we take a treat out. I'm sure that's what she was saying.

June 24—Lorie had a good week. She has been so cooperative with the flannel board and characters. She was jabbering up a storm as she put them up on the board.

End of July—*end of summer school*—Lorie had a good week. Lorie just walks everywhere now. She'll walk out on the grass rather than crawl. Now that she is walking, she puts her napkins in the wastebasket, walks over to shut the door on request, and I am trying to incorporate more simple commands that she can do to help in the room. She seems to enjoy doing them.

A Time of Victories

September 3—Lorie seemed much happier today! [She had to get used to going to school again, as she had a month of vacation.] She kept saying "hi ya" when someone would come in the room. She's quite a greeter. She and Stacy were playing by the mirror today, and it looke like a fun game of peek-a-boo!

September 9—a lot of vocalizing today: "hat," 'bubs" for bubbles, "up", and a lot of jargon-type talking. She was more outgoing today and participated in our activities. [She was feeling bad while cutting an eyetooth.] Lorie was dry and went on the toilet today.

September 15—Lorie was so talkative today: "up," "down," "hat," "sit own" [sit down], "hi ya," "pop." She just seems to be jabbering all day long.

September 23—Lorie got a bite on her left arm today by one of the little boys. It didn't break the skin, but it did leave a mark. [These children do not act differently than normal children.] Lorie got up at group sing and danced with a partner today. She seemed so pleased to do it by herself without someone having to be sure she wouldn't fall. Also, a kitty was at the Center for a short time today, and Lorie said "meow" when she saw it.

September 27—Lorie was a "bossy" little girl today. She was telling everyone what to do: "okay," "sit own," "over there," etc. A real talker today.

October 11—Lorie participated very well in the Rebus Program for a first session. [This is a new speech program they are using.] She tried the sign for "box" three to four times. She sat and watched intently.

The Lorie of today is not a passive child. She is a little girl, growing, developing; she has her own little personality. She is a fighter in trying to overcome parts of her handicap.

In May, the Day Activity Center of our county and one of a neighboring county got together and had a Special Olympics. I went with my Christian friend, Beth. She has a son at the Day Activity Center who is brain damaged. We sat on the grass, enjoyed the beautiful day, and watched all the activities that had been planned for the event.

I wrote an article covering the event for our Retarded Association's local paper:

A VERY SPECIAL OLYMPICS

Shortly after 10 A.M., the Jr. Special Olympics began with several small children running in a foot race. The "go" signal had been sounded and their small bodies darted out, running forward, turning around at the half-way line, and back toward the finish line. The "will to win" could be seen on their small faces, and they continued on with strong determination.

What set this event off from most other contests was the fact that these children, by the world's definition, are handicapped. The events had been geared to their physical abilities.

It was the morning of May 24 and the place for competing was the back yard of the Day Activity Center. The contestants in this Jr. Special Olympics were the small students of the county's two Day Activity Centers. This is a school program set up for mentally handicapped children from the age of two until school age.

The yard was filled with about eighty onlookers who were there either to view or compete in the day's events. It was a lovely, warm, and sunny day. Excitement filled the air as people watched with anticipation. The crowd cheered the small ones on as they went through the events; some of the contestants alone, others with the assistance and encouragement of their parents.

154

The events were varied, and some of the activities were crawling races, running with a cotton ball on a spoon, and finding objects hidden in the corn. Some of the little ones participated in a contest of getting in and out of cardboard boxes.

When all the competition had been completed, a picnic lunch was served. The day's events were completed with the passing out of the awards. Joy and bright smiles could be seen on the little ones' faces when they received a ribbon for winning first or second in one of the contests. And, needless to say, there were a lot of proud parents, too!

With a little hope, encouragement, love, and help, these children showed they were able to compete. There is already talk of another Jr. Special Olympics next year—this one was such a success!

Lorie won a blue ribbon in the crawling race, and was she ever proud of herself! Of course, her mommy was proud, too!

In the spring, Lorie had been in a style show our Down's parents' group put on with our children as the models. I went across the stage with Lorie to help her, and when she saw everyone paying attention, she stopped and became a "ham" for them. The crowd roared—she captured their hearts! And the neat thing about doing this was that we got to keep the outfit Lorie modeled: a cute two-piece, aqua-plaid slacks outfit.

If you were to meet Don and me today, you would find that we are very positive people concerning our daughter. We are always telling people positive things concerning her schooling, past programs, the things she is now doing, plus some of her daily antics. Right now, her latest antics are throwing the contents of a drawer or two around; the other day it was a sheet and pillow case drawer!

We love her and do not feel sorry for ourselves because we did not have a "normal" daughter. And we do not feel sorry for her. We know that God is pouring grace on her to help her make it in this world. Lorie is a fighter; she keeps at things until she masters them. As Chris Byroads, her past music therapist, says, "These children are better fighters than any normal person will ever be!" And she is right. Lorie doesn't give up; she keeps trying and trying until she eventually does it! She is much more determined than her normal brother, who sometimes complains when he can't do something on the first try. I don't think Lorie has the concept of giving up. Maybe her determination is because of her handicap.

Recently God used Don and me in the life of one of my girl friends whose husband walked out on her and their two boys. I have spent much time with her trying to help her through the rough days of rejection and trying to turn her life around. I am amazed by the many things I am able to share with her that the Lord has taught us through Lorie.

I wouldn't have been able to understand or help in my friend's situation unless I had suffered and learned from a sad situation myself. I have been able to show her that God can, indeed, turn her tragedy around, as He has in our case.

Don and I may never know all the reasons why we received Lorie, just as Job in the Bible didn't know why he had to suffer. We are thankful for the reasons He has show us, but it isn't important that we know every single reason why.

We know from the Bible that God was controlling how Lorie was being formed in my womb. He made her the way she is. He could have corrected her birth defect and made her perfect, but He didn't! Lorie being Down's Syndrome is His will for her!

Somehow, knowing that He permitted Lorie to be a

special child and knowing that we do not have to know every reason why has helped us in accepting it.

Our attitude toward our special child does make a difference; our positive attitude can become their positive attitude toward themselves. A positive attitude is important for all of us!

Someone has said, "Mentally retarded people can help, with your help." Lorie can do things if she is helped, and Don and I are doing our best to help her.

The other day at our Down's parents' group we saw a very positive movie on the Down's person from birth until adulthood. We saw the special schooling available for the infant and on up for both the trainable and educable person. These children can be taught to do jobs and can work in either sheltered workshops or at certain jobs. They can live in group homes, and some higher functioning mentally retarded people have been able to get their own apartments. One woman shown in the film works in a cafeteria and manages it alone in the morning while waiting on customers and getting the food ready for the lunch hour. She even orders all the food from the suppliers. She is managing very well in this responsible job.

If there are to be changes in the world for the handicapped person, it has to begin with our concept of them. We are going to have to see them differently; we must see them as persons much like us. They may be slower, blind, or have some other drawback because of their handicap, but they can be a useful part of our world if we give them a chance!

My attitude toward and concept of the handicapped person was based more on feelings than knowledge, until I was forced to seriously think about handicapped people as people. Since then, my thinking concerning handicapped people has completely changed. Isn't it time the world starts seeing them in a different light? The public deserves to have another view besides the stereotypes that are presented in the media and by some in the medical profession.

Handicapped people are not mistakes; they are God's will and He has a unique purpose for them. We recently heard Joni Eareckson speak. She is a beautiful, young woman who is quadriplegic, and she is a good example of how God can use a handicapped person to get His message across. Tears ran down my cheeks as I saw and heard the beautiful testimony she gave to us, and it was evident that God had permitted her to become handicapped.

Another popular quote is, "God doesn't make junk!" How true that is. Lorie isn't junk; she is a special and beautiful person who is teaching us so many special things. She is a little ray of sunshine in our home.

Tonight as I watch my two children—the beautiful gifts God gave Don and me—I see many wonderful things. Kevin has taken out two sheets of paper, and he and Lorie are drawing pictures. How wonderful that God planned Kevin to be Lorie's older brother; he is perfect for her. He is patient and kind and does many things with her. He admires her hair when it is curled, claps when she does something new, and lets her follow him around. She adores her older brother!

This summer we went to visit some friends who live in Wyoming. They told me they did not know much about Down's Syndrome, and they expected Lorie to be a lot different than she is.

This statement sums it up: Handicapped people are different than we expect them to be! Lorie is certainly different from what we were led to believe she would be!

One day my friend Cris asked me, "Do most of the

Down's parents you know rely on Jesus to help them make it?"

"No, I don't know many who are in the Lord."

"How in the world do they make it? How do they cope, manage, and accept it without Jesus?"

"I don't know," I replied. Her question made me think about how they manage without Him. To me, my coming this far in accepting Lorie's handicap has come with Jesus helping me every step of the way. He is continuing to guide me; without Him, I couldn't make it!

Don and I don't know what the future holds for us in rearing Lorie—we only know who is controlling it. And with Him, we can make it through the rough times ahead, as well as the happy times when the victories come.

Some of the victories that have come lately have pleased us. One was just before the fall session when the school physical therapist tested Lorie. Lorie was testing mostly around two years of age. Don and I were very pleased, as there is only a seven-month lag right now, and we do not think this is at all bad. The school speech therapist put Lorie in the highest group in speech. Lorie understands words very well and can say several words. These are happy notes. Lorie, we are told, is doing well in school, and we are thankful.

We are hoping, since Lorie is doing so well in speech, that she will learn how to talk well. If she does, this ability will be a plus for the rest of her life.

Lorie is indeed a special gift the Lord has given us to enjoy, help, and learn from. I can't imagine our life without her.

Our world is changing. We have moved from Minnesota to Illinois, and Don has a better job than he has ever had before. We know that Lorie will have good schooling here. We don't know all the reasons why Jesus has led us here, but He must have a purpose. I hope God will use us to touch people's lives through our accepting Lorie and through Lorie herself. And we believe we have shown our friends in Minneapolis the love of Jesus and what He has done in our lives. I pray that He will continue to use us and show more people His wonderful love, care, concern, and guidance, and that He loves them, too!

We know that God did not give us Lorie to punish us for sins, but to reach us and show us His love for us and to conform us more and more to the image of His Son.

"Mommy, Mommy!" Kevin calls out. "Lorie just dumped Daddy's sock drawer!"

I'm off to pick up the mess—our daughter is not passive. She is a bundle of fun, work, joy, and so many other things wrapped up in a special gift to us. She is our special angel with a bit of mischief added in!

Staying Up With the Down's Syndrome Child

We are handicapped on all sides, but we are never frustrated; we are puzzled, but never in despair. We are persecuted, but we never have to stand it alone: we may be knocked down but we are never knocked out! Every day we experience something of the death of Jesus . . . in these bodies of ours . . . . We wish you could see how all this is working out for your benefit, and how the more grace God gives, the more thanksgiving will redound to his glory. This is the reason we never collapse (2 Corinthians 4:8—10,15,16).*

Some of you who are reading this book may be new parents of a Down's Syndrome baby and may have bought this book to search for some answers to your situation. I hope the things the Lord has taught us have been of help to you.

We know that you have an array of emotions—we

*J.B. Phillips: *The New Testament in Modern English*, revised edition. ©J.B. Phillips 1958, 1960,1972. Used by permission of Macmillan Publishing Co. ,Inc.

161

have been there! Your feelings are probably running havoc from hurt, shock, disappointment, anger, confusion, to many more unnamed emotions.

A feeling is an internal sensation that is an involuntary response to a mental or physical stimulus. A feeling can be pleasurable or painful, but it is neither right nor wrong; it is what we do with it that causes right or wrong responses.

One thing both Don and I recommend is for you to face your feelings—both negative and positive.

Dante Cicchetti, who is now an assistant professor in psychology at Harvard, states this same fact:

> The best thing in the beginning is to be as honest with yourself as you can be in facing your feelings and knowing that it is normal to have them. By being in touch with your emotions, you can then express them to someone you trust. If you delude yourself into thinking everything is rosy or terrible, it will likely affect the whole family. And as you work out your feelings, you are able to adjust.

Facing our feelings is not easy, because we do not like to admit we have negative feelings. But we have these feelings along with good ones, and the sooner we admit them and get them out in the open, the sooner we can face them.

One of the hardest things to admit to people is, "Yes, I am angry this happened to us!" So we usually stuff this reaction down inside, sometimes resulting, as in my case, in depression. But feelings do not stay stuffed down. They sneak back up and cause havoc in our bodies. It's much better to face our anger or whatever feelings and let Jesus help us work through them.

Others of us have been thrust into a world we know little about, and we are concerned about the length of time it will take us to adjust. Since we are all individuals, we adjust differently, according to how willing we are to come to terms with the fact.

I don't think we need to be overly concerned about not adjusting as fast as the next person; the important thing is just to work at facing the situation, feelings, and emotions as soon as possible, and when we do, the adjusting will come.

Don and I have both come to terms with the fact that we will never be completely done with the adjusting process. Up the road, there will always be new things to face and adjust to as we rear our special daughter. We have already faced some different adjustments: when we were first told; Lorie's first days at infant stimulation and music therapy; her being slower physically and starting the D.A.C. Parents whose child has a bad heart or other physical problem have even more continual adjustments to make.

Don and I are starting to adjust to the fact that some people are noticing that Lorie looks "different." We used to go everywhere with Lorie, and no one gave us a second glance. Now this is changing. People will first look at Lorie, then at us, and back to Lorie, all the time giving us odd looks. We are trying to act as normally as possible with Lorie while this is going on. And we often smile at them, and this causes a surprised reaction in them.

It is important that you see your child as an individual—it's important not only for *your* adjustment, but for your child's adjustment. As Dante says, "It is important to give the Down's child, as any other child, the idea that he or she is a unique and different individual who has his own personality and feelings." God has made our special children as distinct and different as we all are.

It is easy for us to focus on ourselves when we have a

special child, but what about our child? God does permit us to have these children as a means of drawing us to Him and teaching us to trust Him, but we must be careful not to focus on this aspect so much that we do not consider our child. Remember, God gave us our children with the responsibility of rearing them, and we have even more responsibility with a special child. And our children have a right to have their needs met.

Repeating what Chris Byroads says, "Rearing these children is a special challenge." And it is! But the rewards are super; the excitement when they master a task is really something, and you do not take anything for granted with them. A warm and loving home for them makes a difference.

"With the handicapped child, you aren't going to prove any points," Chris continues. "If they overcome their handicap, it proves human nature will overcome to survive. With a handicapped child, you are done with the status symbols. Everything you once thought was important before, ninety-eight percent of it will go. The truth comes down to either you love or don't love your child, and if you do, you will do anything to help your child to have the happiest life possible. In our day, people don't try for a happy life; they are trying for a productive and successful life."

We have elected to keep Lorie, because we love her and feel that a loving home is the best place for her. We want to assure her of the best possible start toward a happy life. So many things we once thought were important have not been since she arrived; our whole concept of what is important has changed.

For you to start the ball rolling in doing something for your special child, I can give you some helpful suggestions. First of all, you can contact the Association of Retarded Citizens (if there is one in your area), or you can call the public health nurse to see if she has any information. If both of these draw "no's," you can then write to:

NARC (National Association for Retarded Children)
2709 Avenue E., East
Arlington, Texas 76010

American Association on Mental Deficiency
6201 Connecticut Avenue
Washington, D.C. 20015

Council for Exceptional Children
1411 Jefferson Davis Highway
Arlington, Virginia 22202

"You know," Chris Byroads told me one day, "Don's reaction to Lorie's being handicapped was unusual."

"What do you mean?" I asked.

"His accepting the fact right away was not typical. If there's anyone who won't accept a child's being handicapped, it usually is the father."

As time goes on, both Don and I have seen situations where this is true, and it makes us feel sad. A husband's strong support and acceptance are important for his wife and family. If any of you fathers out there are having a hard time in this area, please remember God put you as head of your family, and your family needs you to be the strong support. Your acceptance is important! It's hard to swallow your pride and humble yourself to accept this, but really, it's for the best. You are hurting your whole family if you do not come to terms with this situation—plus, you are rebelling against God's will for your life. Ask God to lead you in this area.

If you know parents of a Down's Syndrome child, do

not be afraid to call them or go over for a visit. You will find they can be helpful and can share various things from having their special child. And getting to know other Down's parents and their children is beneficial—it's nice to know someone in your same situation.

Most parents of Down's children have strong feelings about conveying a realistic concept to the world concerning the Down's Syndrome individual. When this subject came up once, Dante's reply was, "No one person or group is going to totally change things."

I asked him, "Do you think you can do more in educating the public now that you have your doctorate?"

"I will be in a better position to help make some changes come about by the results of my research and our future book. It will help having professional people read the results," was his reply.

We parents would like to rear our special children as normally as possible, but how can we best do this? Is keeping them home, withholding therapy programs, and not attending support groups giving them as normal a life as possible?

I have heard people say that they do not want to bring their child to programs, because they do not want their child to be exposed to other retarded children. They are afraid their child will pick up some of the "awful" traits these retarded children have. In all the time I was taking Lorie to group therapy, I never saw any of these so-called "bad" traits that they are afraid of.

Or they say, "I do not need to go to parents' or mothers' groups. I don't need them or their silly visiting!"

These support groups help parents in adjusting and in all the other things that crop up while rearing a special child. People there can share common experiences, how they handled various situations, plus give a bounty of useful information. Some of the group events we attended included educational programs or discussions of subjects important to us parents. One time we learned where we could obtain insurance for our special children. This is not an easy thing do to!

I often sense that the person who says he does not need to attend support sessions is really saying, "I am a self-sufficient person, and going there would be the same as saying I need to have someone help me." They don't like to admit they can't handle this situation perfectly! As I mentioned before, having a special child humbles you. You find out you will have to rely on many people to help you as you rear him or her.

This doesn't make you less of a person. In many ways, it tones down pride and helps you learn to receive aid from others. In turn you can help parents who need counsel and encouragement. Don and I know so little about all that is involved in rearing Lorie, and we are always thankful for any help we receive.

It has been banding together (especially in Associations for Retarded Citizens) of parents who have been fighting for changes that enables special children to have a more normal life. Parents of these children have fought for public schooling for handicapped children, for mainstreaming whenever possible, for group homes, sheltered workshops, and a host of other things that our children can benefit from.

Parents years earlier fought for the Day Activity Center that Lorie was able to enjoy. What can we do for other parents to help make the future better for their special children? And what can we do for our child's future?

You do not have to join every group, or even attend them constantly. Don and I were attending a once-every-two-months parent's group, and I went alone to the D.A.C. mothers' group whenever I could. I did not go the mothers' group every week while writing this book, but when I did attend I enjoyed visiting with the moms and being part of the interesting group conversations that occurred while I was there. I'm glad there are understanding people and help for us.

So how do we rear our special children as normally as possible? First of all, we must give them all the help they need. Therapy helps the special child function in our world. Children who have therapy are able to walk, talk, and do all kinds of things sooner than those without this advantage. This, in turn, helps them function not that much differently from normal children, especially in the early years. And although the differences increase between them and their normal peers as they get older, special children can still be taught to function in jobs and do other useful things to insure a purposeful life.

Before Dante left Minneapolis, he commented about Lorie: "One of the things I have noticed about Lorie, from as far back as I can remember, is that she always seems to be interested in solving the problems we give her to do, and she takes enjoyment in doing them. Lorie seems to improve with age and especially in her gross and fine motor development. I have seen all along a higher degree of perseverance and a lot of 'expressability' in her problem solving. We think these strides are good, since having the motivation to solve problems may help her out later as things get tougher and tougher."

Linda, Dante's assistant, has gone to Massachusetts to do her graduate work in clinical psychology. She had been in one of Dante's classes studying the development of atypical children when Dante had asked for volunteers for his research program.

Linda told us the last time we saw her: "I always enjoyed coming out to see Lorie for the 'Laugh and Smile' part. We found time to talk with you while playing with Lorie. The hardest part of our job was communicating to you parents all the unusual things we wanted you to do to make the babies laugh, especially walking like Charlie Chaplin, which was the most hated item on the list! I admire mothers like you for putting up with us every time we came out. And getting to know you parents and the children is something I will remember all my life."

Chris Byroads left our life too; her husband was transferred, and they moved to Kansas. Chris was important in my life, and she helped me tremendously. I'm thankful for all she did for me.

We have been grateful (God has had His hand in this area) about Lorie's health. The only serious thing she has ever had was the start of pneumonia. Since some of you reading this book may have a child with physical problems, I will give you my friend Sue's story, because her Down's Syndrome son has heart problems.

Sue and Doug had two normal sons when their third son, Stevie, arrived and was diagnosed Down's Syndrome. It was a shock to Sue, even though she was already in the Lord: "I had been in a time of seeking my own will and not the Lord's, and it was a time where my faith seemed to be lagging. I had prayed for a normal baby (my will), but it was not the Lord's will. He had a different plan for my life, which included a special child. God has used this situation to help my growth and to open my eyes to the world of the retarded."

Sue's story begins in the hospital when Stevie was first born, and he turned blue twelve hours later. "They told me after they put him in a warmer that it could be a sign of heart problems."

The doctor was concerned and immediately had Stevie X-rayed. His heart looked okay. The doctor told Doug and Sue that a heart problem may or may not show up later on.

When Stevie was a month old, Sue started noticing that he was breathing rapidly and that he did not have a strong sucking motion. As he was drinking his bottle, his forehead would be full of beads of perspiration. The doctor discovered a heart murmur when Stevie was two months old.

X rays taken when Stevie was four months old showed an enlarged heart, and Doug and Sue were told that Stevie was in heart failure. This was causing him to be weak and constantly exhausted.

Sue worried a lot about his physical condition. He gained only six pounds the first year of his life and weighed twelve pounds on his first birthday. At about nine months, he seemed to be sick all the time with colds, viruses, and other things that he didn't seem to be able to shake. Sue was having a hard time feeding him, as he spit it back or choked on whatever she gave him.

At eleven-and-a-half months, Doug and Sue were becoming more and more concerned, as Stevie seemed to be turning bluer after baths and his heartbeat was up, although not all the time. They went back to the heart specialist, and he told them that Stevie wasn't any worse, but that he wasn't very good. He decided to do a heart catheterization to determine whether Stevie would need surgery and to see where the holes in the heart were.

This was done when Stevie was twelve-and-a-half months old, and he was put in the hospital for two days. Doug and Sue were told that Stevie had a large hole in the center of his heart, which involved all four chambers. He also had two defective valves. This was causing a great amount of pressure from the excess blood flowing to his lungs. A banding was going to have to be done to prevent lung damage, for which, they were told, there was no cure.

The doctors wanted the surgery performed right away, and just before it was to take place, Stevie got pneumonia, and the operation had to be postponed. A month later he had his surgery, which consisted of putting a band around the pulmonary artery to restrict the excess flow of blood to the lungs.

As the result of his surgery, Stevie is doing well and has gotten up to a normal weight for him. "The last time we saw the doctor," Sue told me, "he said the difference in the way Stevie is now from the way he was before the banding is a miracle.

"When the time for his banding surgery came," Sue continued, "I almost chickened out and wanted to cancel the surgery. We were then told Stevie hadn't a choice, as he was using up his energy just lying in his crib. Doug and I did not have a choice either; we had to give our son over to God's care and trust Him with the outcome.

"We both came to terms with the fact that God gave us Stevie with these problems, and since He doesn't make mistakes, we knew that Stevie had been given to us for our good. And we knew that Jesus had a purpose in this, even if we had Stevie only for a short time.

"We said a prayer to God turning Stevie over to Him—the fear was still there and we didn't know the outcome, but we were calmer and had more strength to handle the situation.

"I learned to change my priorities around and really depend on Jesus. We knew that we had to give not only Stevie over to His care, but our two normal sons as well. We all really belong to Him."

Lorie

Stevie will have surgery between the ages of four and seven to correct his heart problems.

Parents of special children often fear losing them. The story of my girl friend, Gail, follows, telling of the time she had to come to terms with this possibility.

It was a rough time for Gail and Bob; they had just come home with a new baby daughter when their Down's Syndrome daughter had to be put into the hospital with pneumonia, and it was touch and go for Stacie's making it. Gail took it hard and cried a lot. Bob was starting to realize that they should put Stacie in God's hands.

"It was my brother who really got us to do something," Gail told me, "when he asked us if we could put Stacie in God's hands and trust Him with the outcome. It wasn't easy, but we said the prayer with him. Immediately afterward, I felt strength pouring through me, and I went home calmer than I had been in days. I was even able to talk to people about Stacie's problems without breaking into tears. I think in this time God used me to be a witness in my sister's life."

Stacie started getting better and was soon home with her brother and sister. It wasn't the Lord's will to take her, but He had asked her parents to trust Him with the outcome.

When it comes down to incidents such as the last two, what really matters? This life is fleeting, and we do not have a lot of time here. Isn't it at times like these that we see how important Jesus is and that He is the only answer to today's problems?

If Jesus is not your Savior, I hope you will consider Him. He is knocking on the door of your heart, and you have only to let Him in. Jesus loves and cares for you, and He can help you rear this special child. You do not have to go the road alone! The choice is yours.

To Friends and Relatives of
Down's Syndrome Children

I think one of the hardest areas for you friends and relatives to deal with is what to do or say when you first find out about the birth of a handicapped child. Maybe you, too, are thrown into a world you know little about, and you are trying to cope with the news, also. Again, I would recommend you face your feelings right away, especially you relatives. The family needs to know you care for them and accept this newest addition to the family.

Many people have a tendency to stay away from the hospital because they do not know what to say; this is a mistake. Relatives and friends who take this route make the parents feel ignored or rejected. You do not have to say a brilliant speech; in fact, you don't have to say anything. Your going there says more than words; it tells the parents that you care.

The parents may or may not talk a lot to you about their special child and how they are feeling. You can do a lot to reassure them of your desire to help, and you can be a good listener.

In the paper one day there was a letter asking if a person should buy a baby gift for a child born with Down's Syndrome. Why not? Don't they think this child is a baby? Of course you take gifts! This child needs clothes, diapers, and all the things any baby needs. And your gift reassures the parents that you care about their baby.

Also, remember to continue showing concern after the mother and baby have gone home. They still need much support during their initial time of adjustment. Some people rally around the parents in the beginning and then forget them later on. Continued support is important.

Lorie

Recently a friend of mine came for a visit. She had a question to ask me and wanted to know if she had done the right thing.

"Mary Ann," she began, "I just went to see a mother and her new baby daughter. When I was holding the baby, I noticed the same Down's Syndrome characteristics that I noticed in Lorie when she was small. The mother didn't say anything to me about the possibility; in fact, she acted as if her baby was perfect. I didn't say anything. Did I do the right thing?"

I felt that she had done the right thing, as with the baby being so small, there is a chance the doctor hadn't discovered the handicap, and if he had, maybe he hadn't told the parents yet. You certainly do not want to be the person to blow it. And if the mother knew, maybe she was not ready to tell people, as it was still too new to her and she was trying to accept it.

It may be a different story if the baby is much older and the parents don't know. Most of the time, however, it is just best to wait until the parents are willing to tell others, and sometimes that takes time.

Don and I met a couple whose daughter is four months old, and the doctor suspected she might have Down's Syndrome. I, wanting to show this new couple a positive outlook, told them about the good programs for Down's children, how well Lorie is doing, and so on. I must have scared the poor mother, who hadn't adjusted to knowing her child might be Down's Syndrome, and she ran off crying. I had blown it, and I felt ashamed.

I need to remember that new parents are not where I am, and it is best to go slowly with them. It takes time to adjust, cope, and accept the situation. I learned another lesson.

Maybe someday the woman I upset will look back at our conversation and think, "Those parents have a

Down's Syndrome daughter, and they don't think it's the worst thing in the world!"

Dante has a good comment for professional people who deal in our lives right after our special child is born. He says, "Parents face a great disappointment when they realize their baby is going to be different from what they had expected. When their encounters with both professional and lay people are insensitive, it only adds to their grief and uncertainty."

Donald and I are strong believers in rearing our special child at home. We know that she functions better in a loving home, and by keeping her here she has a chance of a higher I.Q.

We are trying to rear Lorie normally, and we expect her to do certain things, just as we expect her brother to do things. We are now working on teaching her limitations in what she can and cannot touch—lots of fun! She really isn't that much different than her brother, just slower.

Don and I still can't understand why, when a child isn't born normal, medical people recommend giving these children up? These children need loving parents just as any other child does. Why deny them their parents' love?

Handicapped children can function very well at home, since most of them are not severely retarded— most have I.Q.'s between forty-five and fifty-four. Parents can manage very well with them at home. I know there are extreme cases where it is not feasible to keep the child at home, but for almost all of us, there is no reason why we can't take care of our special child.

The choice of giving the child up or keeping him or her in the hospital should not be offered to parents right away. After first learning of the baby's handicap, parents are so emotionally upset that they cannot make a decision very well. It's better to take the child home and try. Every one that I know of who has taken his child home, has not been sorry and would not give up his child for the world.

And today, the many programs to help the retarded are making it possible for us to rear our children at home without a tremendous financial burden. And as mentioned previously, there are parent groups that offer help and support.

Really, when you give up your child without trying, who is first, you or the child? I'm sure my remarks will not settle well with some, but this is how we feel. This was the Lord's will for our lives, and I'm sure He expects us to grow and learn through rearing this child He gave us. And since God does not give us anything we cannot handle, He knows that we can make it with our child.

So, if you are deciding what to do, take your child home and try. He or she will grow on you. Lorie is a happy child who lives to please us. She has a more positive, happy outlook than most of us. She has captured the hearts of our friends, relatives, and acquaintances. I am so glad God gave her to us!

And last, but not least, Jesus is the answer in our lives and the one who is making us able to rear this special child. He has led and is leading us every step of the way.

Praise the Lord for all He has done in our lives and for what He will continue to do. He is the answer to all of today's problems!

Grandma's Page

Lorie is smiles.
She tenders them to the world
From an inexhaustible supply.
Shy smiles. Questioning ones.
Friendly smiles.
An offering from a happy heart.

Who is Lorie?
A tiny blonde elf
Who gleefully claps her hands
At the antics of this show-off,
Crazy old world.

Music. The world's universal language.
Lorie listens in delight.
And sways in rhythm—
In tune with all time.

—Irma H. Klock

Notes

[1]June Mater, *Make the Most of Your Baby* (Arlington, Texas: National Association for Retarded Citizens, 1974).

[2]David Pitt, *Your Down's Syndrome Child: You Can Help Him Develop From Infancy to Adulthood* (Arlington, Texas: National Association for Retarded Citizens, 1974).

[3]Lucille Poor, *Aim to Fight Low Expectation of Down's Syndrome Children* (Forest Lake, Minnesota: Forest Lake Printing, Inc., 1976), pp. 29,30.

[4]*Ibid.*, p. 70.

[5]*Ibid.*, pp. 5,7.

[6]Dante Cicchetti and A. Sroufe, "The Emotional Development of the Infant With Down's Syndrome," *Aim to Fight Low Expectation of Down's Syndrome Children*, (Forest Lake, Minnesota: Forest Lake Printing, Inc., 1976), pp. 50,51.

Recommended Reading

Educational

Horrobin, J. Margaret, and John E. Rynders. *To Give an Edge*. Obtained by writing to:
    To Give an Edge
    c/o The Colwell Press, Inc.
    500 South Seventh Street
    Minneapolis, Minnesota 55415

The cost is approximately $2.50

Mater, June. *Make the Most of Your Baby*. Arlington, Texas: The National Association for Retarded Citizens, 1974. May be obtained from your local Association for Retarded Citizens or by writing to:
    The National Association for Retarded Citizens
    2709 Avenue E, East
    Arlington, Texas 76010

Pitt, David. *Your Down's Syndrome Child: You Can Help Him Develop From Infancy to Adulthood*. Arlington, Texas: The National Association for Retarded Citizens.

Poor, Lucille. *Aim to Fight Low Expectation of Down's Syndrome Children.* Obtained by writing to:
>   The North Central Publishing Company
>   274 Fillmore Avenue East
>   St. Paul, Minnesota 55107

The cost is $3.95 plus postage.

Practical Advice to Parents: A Guide to Finding Help for Handicapped Children and Youth. Obtained by writing to:
>   The National Information Center for Handicapped
>   P.O. Box 1492
>   Washington D.C. 20013

Sharing Our Caring. This magazine is published five times a year and is written especially for parents of Down's Syndrome children. A year's subscription is $3.50 and can be obtained by writing to:
>   Caring
>   P.O. Box 400
>   Milton, Washington 98354

Christian

Dobson, James. *Hide and Seek.* Old Tappan, N.J.: Fleming H. Revell Co., 1974. This book discusses the importance of self-esteem.

Eareckson, Joni. *Joni.* Grand Rapids, Mich.: Zondervan Publishing House, 1976. This is the story of a young woman's acceptance of her quadriplegic status and her victory over depression.

Evans, Dale. *Angel Unaware.* Westwood, N.J.: Fleming

H. Revell Co., 1953. Recommended reading after your child is a few months old.

LaHaye, Tim. *How to Win Over Depression*. Grand Rapids, Mich.: Zondervan Publishing House, 1974.

Landorf, Joyce. *The Mourning Song*. Old Tappan, N.J.: Fleming H. Revell Co., 1974.

Nason, Michael, and Donna Nason. *Tara: The Dramatic Story of a Brain Injured Child's Courageous Fight to Get Well*. New York: Hawthorn Books, 1976.

Schultz, Edna Moore. *Kathy*. Chicago: Moody Press, 1963. A story about a Down's Syndrome girl.

Swindoll, Charles R. *You and Your Child*. Nashville: Thomas Nelson Inc., Publishers, 1977. Note especially the chapter entitled, "The Handicapped Child," pp. 132–135.